American Cancer Society
PROSTATE CANCER

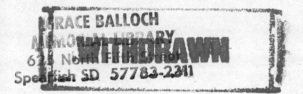

ALSO BY
THE AMERICAN CANCER SOCIETY

WOMEN AND CANCER

COLORECTAL CANCER

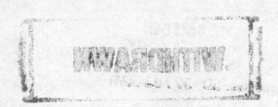

American Cancer Society

PROSTATE CANCER

What Every Man—and His Family—Needs to Know

REVISED AND UPDATED

David G. Bostwick, M.D.

Gregory T. MacLennan, M.D.

Thayne R. Larson, M.D.

Editorial Project Director

Ron Schaumburg

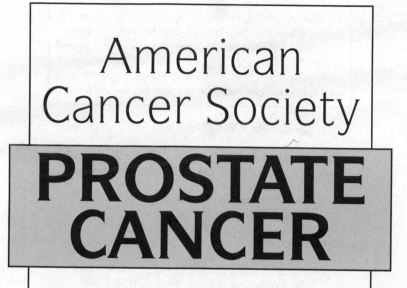

VILLARD • NEW YORK

Copyright © 1996, 1999 by The American Cancer Society

All rights reserved under International and Pan-American Copyright Conventions. Published in the United States by Villard Books, a division of Random House, Inc., New York, and simultaneously in Canada by Random House of Canada Limited, Toronto.

VILLARD BOOKS and colophon are registered trademarks of Random House, Inc.

This is a revised edition of *Prostate Cancer*, published in 1996 by Villard Books, a division of Random House, Inc.

The table on page 68 is reproduced by permission of the American Urological Association.

Illustrations copyright © 1996 Mayo Clinic. Used by permission.

Library of Congress Cataloging-in-Publication Data
Bostwick, David G.
Prostate cancer : what every man—and his family—needs to know /
David G. Bostwick, Gregory T. MacLennan, Thayne R. Larson: editorial project director, Ron Schaumburg.
p.   cm.
At head of title: The American Cancer Society.
Includes bibliographical references and index.
ISBN 0-375-75319-2
1. Prostate—Cancer—Popular works.   I. MacLennan, Gregory T.
II. Larson, Thayne R.   III. Schaumburg, Ron.   IV. American Cancer Society.   V. Title.
RC280.P7B67   1996
616.99'463—dc20   96-8588

Random House website address: www.atrandom.com
Printed in the United States of America on acid-free paper
2 4 6 8 9 7 5 3
Revised and Updated Edition

To my family—always cheerfully patient with my distractedness. Kathleen, Daniel, and Brian—thanks for your love and good humor. And to my wife, Betsy, deep thanks for your apparently bottomless well of support, advice, warmth, and love.

—DGB

To my family—my wife, Carrol, and my sons, Darren and Grayden, in appreciation of your unswerving loyalty, support, and understanding during my years of training and during the production of this book.

—GTM

To my wife, Carol Ann, and my children, Benjamin, Mia, Claire, and Nathan, for your unstinting love, support, and encouragement. I also dedicate this book to my hundreds of patients and their spouses, who over the years have taught me more than any book or school could. In living with and managing prostate cancer, they demonstrate on a daily basis what heroism truly means.

—TRL

Foreword

by Jim Mullen
Founder, Man to Man

My life changed forever when, more than a decade ago, a doctor told me I had prostate cancer. At first I was shocked and confused. I didn't know what the prostate was; had never even heard the word before. If my wife, Marian, had not insisted I see the doctor to find out why I'd been urinating so often, I might never have known about this tiny, troublesome gland.

The doctor wanted to stretch me out on the table and carve me up the next day. But Marian insisted we get a second opinion. The next doctor thought I was too old for surgery—although sixty-eight didn't seem that old to me—and he recommended radiation.

In my generation, we were brought up to rely on our doctors 100 percent. We thought M.D. stood for *medical deity*. But here I'd gotten two completely different stories from two different specialists. That was just the beginning. In the months that followed I had a lot of trouble finding out what was happening to my body, what choices I had, what my long-term prospects were. I needed more help and information than I was getting.

So I went to a local hospital and sat in on a meeting of one of their cancer support groups. Most of the participants were women. There were a few other guys there with prostate conditions, but we all sat there like bumps on a log. None of us did any talking. Afterwards, I asked one of them, "Why didn't you ask any questions about your prostate?" He looked surprised and said, "Not in front of those women!"

That night I told Marian what had happened. I said I felt like I'd run up against a brick wall. She said simply, "Why don't you start your own group?" So I called the other fellows and invited them to the house for coffee, cookies, and a chance to talk about our common problem. That meeting, in the kitchen of our Sarasota home, was the start of Man to Man, now a nationwide support group for prostate cancer survivors.

That was back in the Dark Ages, at least in terms of prostate cancer awareness, when even though hundreds of thousands of men developed the disease each year and tens of thousands died from it, prostate cancer was like a big, dark secret.

It's not a secret anymore. Today there's a worldwide movement to educate men about the disease. Newspapers and television shows discuss the subject openly. Community programs spread the word about the importance of screening tests and annual examinations. Patient support networks spread the word about the latest developments. The American Cancer Society is playing a leadership role, not only through its ongoing research into the treatment and prevention of prostate cancer, but also through its public education efforts. The book you are holding in your hands is part of that outreach.

In obvious ways, prostate cancer is an exclusively male problem. Of course, men are the only ones who get the disease. But male psychology plays a big part as well.

During my life I've spent a lot of time in the company of men. I was cocaptain of the University of Delaware football team in 1941, the year the team celebrated its first undefeated season. I served as an officer in the Marine Corps in World War II and was wounded on Iwo Jima. From the gridiron to the battlefield to the workplace jungle, I have seen men face incredible challenges and come through with flying colors.

When faced with a life-threatening medical problem, though, a lot of guys drop the ball. Some are just plain scared of doctors. They're afraid of knives or needles—or a doctor's probing finger. Some feel that if they get sick, their only option is to "be a man" and tough it out. Stoically, they refuse to let anyone know that they are suffering. They keep their thoughts and feelings locked up inside and refuse to ask for, let alone accept, any help. When they find out that prostate cancer threatens their erections or their urinary control, they feel that the very essence of their manhood is being threatened. Some adopt a macho stance—"Cut this critter out of me!"—without considering other measures that might produce results that are just as good. Or they put off making a decision, refusing to make a move until they can be absolutely sure of doing the right thing. By that time, it may be too late.

Prostate cancer is not just a man's problem: It has a profound effect on wives and families as well. There is enormous emotional, financial, and physical stress in dealing with a life-threatening disease. The sexual impact can cause a man to withdraw from his partner, robbing a couple of precious intimacy and closeness. And coping with side effects of treatment can cause the family to retreat from friends and society.

This book, written by three leading experts in the field, gives straightforward medical information about prostate cancer and its treatment. It also presents the steps you need to take in making some tough choices, and directs you to valuable resources for more information. There are also helpful first-hand accounts from men and women around the country, veterans of the battle against prostate cancer.

The situation today is very different from the one I encountered just a few years ago. More and more people are taking charge of their health care. They realize that doctors don't have all the answers, and so they do their own digging. They're learning the value of speaking up and speaking out, of being active partners in their treatment. They demand to know all the options open to them. And men are more willing to join forces with other men and couples to seek answers—and share what they discover.

In the fight against prostate cancer, such sharing is powerful medicine.

SARASOTA, FLORIDA
MARCH 1996

Foreword

by Henry A. Porterfield
Chairman, US TOO International, Inc.

Each day in this country, nearly a thousand men find out they have prostate cancer. I am proud to serve as chairman of US TOO, an international network of prostate cancer survivors. Our motto is "Learning to cope through knowledge and hope." Those few words sum up everything that is important about dealing with a serious but treatable medical condition. It also reflects the purpose of this book.

Learning to cope with prostate cancer means many things. On one level, it means navigating your way through a medical maze: talking with doctors, making sense of the information, and exerting a strong voice in the choice of treatment. It means coping with the long-term issues, such as the side effects of treatment. Coping also means addressing the emotional and psychological impact of prostate cancer, an issue not just for the man with the condition but for his wife and his family as well.

Knowledge is an essential tool for effective coping. The mission of US TOO is to make the facts available and to help survivors understand their situation. We use all the means at our disposal. Besides offering lectures and workshops at group meetings, we sponsor a newsletter, publish pamphlets, run a telephone hotline, and develop educational outreach programs. In this book you will find the information you need to understand your cancer and what the different treatments involve.

But facts by themselves are not enough. A man with prostate cancer also needs hope — to know that treatments work, that problems can be managed, that life does go on. Hope comes from the reports in the scientific literature of discoveries about the nature of prostate cancer and promising new ways to combat it. Hope comes from the outspokenness of prostate cancer survivors — among them such noted figures as Senator Bob Dole, General Norman Schwarzkopf, and the actors Sidney Poitier and Robert Goulet — who are willing to spread the word about the importance of early detection and treatment. Most of all, hope is found in the eyes, the voices, and the smiles of the men who have been down that road.

Since its founding in 1990 as a not-for-profit organization administered for and by prostate cancer survivors, US TOO has developed into an international volunteer movement with more than 400 chapters here and abroad. Each year, our 60,000 members and another 100,000 of their family members and friends benefit from our close ties to the medical community. We offer a forum where men and women can learn the latest news about prostate cancer and its treatment, compare experiences, and discuss matters of concern. Our goal is to inform the newly diagnosed man about his treatment choices, to support the recently treated man as he anticipates the consequences of therapy, and to help the posttreatment man continue to live the fullest and most rewarding life possible.

When they learn about their diagnosis, many men with prostate cancer feel they have lost control of their lives. They must cope not just with the bewildering external world of medicine, but with the impact on their inner world as well: changes in the status of their health and vitality and in their deepest sense of themselves as men. In our culture, that's not easy for a man to do. There are few opportunities to talk about deeply intimate and personal concerns. To address that need, US TOO maintains an extensive database of information, including the names of survivors who volunteer as counselors and guides — the proverbial shoulders to lean on in times of crisis. However they are structured or run, support groups can dramatically convey the message that, with help from professionals and fellow patients, it is possible for a man with prostate cancer to regain control.

Many of the patients who tell their stories in this book are members of US TOO or other support groups. They are the living embodiment of the philosophy that is part of our organization's logo: "Sharing is caring." By sharing the burden of prostate cancer, the load becomes lighter for everyone.

Hinsdale, Illinois
March 1996

Acknowledgments

During the preparation of this volume we are pleased and proud to have had the support of the American Cancer Society. The book reflects their deep and ongoing commitment to educating people about prostate cancer. We are especially indebted to Dr. Hugh Shingleton, vice president of the American Cancer Society National Home Office in Atlanta, whose unwavering enthusiasm, support, and encouragement inspired all of us.

Special thanks are due to many people who assisted us at various stages of this project. At its inception, the idea was vigorously supported by members of the Prostate Cancer Advisory Board of the American Cancer Society, including Dr. Gerald Murphy, former president of the American Cancer Society and director of the Pacific Northwest Research Foundation, Seattle, Washington; Dr. Reginald Ho, Honolulu, Hawaii, former president of the American Cancer Society; Dr. Harmon Eyre, vice president of the American Cancer Society; Dr. Andrew von Eschenbach, chairman of urology, M. D. Anderson Cancer Center, Houston, Texas. Also, Dr. Michael Brawer; Dr. F. K. Mostofi; Dr. Daniel Miller; Dr. George Jones; Dr. Fred Lee; Dr. Sam Graham, Jr.; Dr. Carl Mansfield; Dr. Gerald Mueller; Dr. Edson Pontes; Dr. Joseph Smith; Dr. Louis Snitkoff; Dr. Harold Amos; Dr. Charles Eytel; Dr. Michael Franklin; Dr. Archie Alexander; Dr. Curtis Mettlin; Dr. Paula Nelson-Marten; and Mr. Leslie Misrock.

We acknowledge the help and encouragement of Dr. George Farrow, Mayo Clinic Department of Pathology, and Dr. David Patterson, Mayo Clinic Department of Urology, who made it possible to collaborate on this project; Dr. Todd Igle, for advice on cryosurgery; and Drs. Gordon Grado and Robert Ferrigni of Mayo Clinic, Scottsdale, Arizona, for their firsthand contribution to the research for this book.

Thanks to Stephen P. Graepel, M.A., of the Mayo Clinic art department for his prompt and professional production of the illustrations.

Thanks to the following individuals: Jim Mullen and Henry A. Porterfield for their forewords; Barbara Lowenstein of Lowenstein and Associates, the project's literary agent, and her staff, especially Norman Kurz; Annik La Farge, our editor at Villard Books; Patty Romanowski, for her work in editing the manuscript; Sybil Pincus, the production editor; Louise Masurat, the copy editor; Rosemarie D. Perrin, Betty Merriman, Greta Durr, Keith Fitzgerald, Terri Ades, and Trish Greene of the American Cancer Society; The American Urological Association and Suzanne Boland Pope; Bob Evans, Margot Fisher, and Susan Paul Schaumburg for their role in editorial development; Gabriela Ferrero for transcription assistance; Annette Bjorheim, Dr. Bostwick's secretary, who coped with this project with her usual efficiency and amiability; and Bud Clarke and Sandy Choron for support and timely advice.

Finally, we must also acknowledge other contributors to this book whose participation has proved enormously valuable. As doctors, we tend to focus on the disease we're treating. As pathologists, we peer through the microscope, studying the defective cells that are threatening someone's life. Caught up as we are in the disease and its progression, at times we may forget to look at our patients as *people*—people whose entire lives are affected physically, emotionally, and spiritually by their condition. To better see the subject from the patient's point of view, we contacted over one hundred men from around the country with prostate cancer, as well as many of their wives and adult children. Through personal interviews, electronic mail, and surveys, we have tried to develop a better sense of the issues that men and their families wrestle with as they struggle to overcome this disease.

We want to acknowledge the courage and generosity of these survivors. Their influence is reflected throughout this book in the personal anecdotes they've shared with us and in the emphasis we have placed on the value of mutual support. By choosing to take control of their lives, these individuals are the real experts in prostate cancer, and they have contributed enormously to the chapters that follow. While some preferred anonymity, those who allowed their names to be used are Don Alonso, Arthur and Susan Bass, George Bateson, Adrian Boie, Steve Corman, Murray H. Corwin, Bill Dehn, Walter Elsaesser, Jim and Ruth Fankhauser, Jim Fulks, Betty Gallo, Joan Kinter, Harry B. Harris, Art Hoffman, Ralph Horvath, Bob and Mavis Immegart, Kent Leach, Dick and Jacquie Lee, Jim Lisec, Urho (Richard) and Ruth Mark, Edwin Megargee and Sara Jill Mercer, DeWitt Ober, Bob Owens, Tony Romao, Bob Samuels, Archie Sanchez, Virgil Simons, Jack Taylor, S. J. Tompkins, Burt Udelson, Manuel Vasquez, Vic Walker, John and Ruth Watford, and William Worrel. Although the patient stories in this book are drawn from interviews, in some cases the anecdotes are composites of experiences from several individuals; details may have been changed and fictional names may be used. No association between any story and the names above should be inferred.

Thanks to Larry and April Becker for their efforts on behalf of the Side by Side support group in Scottsdale, Arizona, and for organizing a special focus group to help the authors plan the book. Thanks, too, to the couples who volunteered to take part in that session and to Ralph Valle, a prostate cancer survivor who helped orchestrate the e-mail portion of the research.

Special thanks to Ron Schaumburg, our hardworking and indefatigable editorial advisor and project director, whose efforts were essential for the timely completion and success of the book.

Contents

Introduction

Each year in this country, more than 317,000 men are found to have cancer in the prostate gland. That is a higher rate than any other cancer in men, including lung and colon cancer, and it outpaces the incidence of breast cancer in women by about 33 percent. Approximately one out of every ten men will develop prostate cancer during his lifetime. Prostate cancer causes more than 41,000 deaths annually—one every thirteen minutes.

But such abstract numbers probably don't mean much to you. When it comes down to it, there is really only one case of prostate cancer that's important, and that's the one you and your family are dealing with right now. Fortunately, as you'll learn in this book, men are living longer with prostate cancer than ever before, and there are many effective treatments that can cure or control the disease.

If you are like most men, receiving a diagnosis of prostate cancer has made you feel as if your life is spinning out of control. Suddenly you are forced to deal with an intimidating health care system as you come to grips with a mysterious and serious disease. You are being asked to make choices that may profoundly affect the quality of the rest of your life.

Our goal in this book is to provide you with the facts you need, the answers you seek, and the support you deserve to help you regain your sense of control.

THE CHALLENGE OF PROSTATE CANCER

Coping with any life-threatening illness poses enormous challenges on many levels: physical, psychological, emotional, and financial. Prostate cancer is an especially troublesome condition for many reasons.

Myths and Misunderstandings

Until recently, the general feeling among the medical community was that prostate cancer was just an "old man's disease" that struck men who would probably die of something else. Such an attitude no longer prevails. We now know that for men in their forties and fifties, prostate cancer is prevalent and deadly—second only to lung cancer as a cause of cancer-related deaths among men—but it is also highly treatable and often curable.

Location of the Prostate in the Body

Because the prostate is buried deep in the pelvis, surrounded by so many other organs and tissues, it can be hard for doctors to determine what is happening there. We have yet to develop foolproof nonsurgical diagnostic techniques. And when cancer is discovered and treated, the prostate's position increases the risk that other organs, such as the bladder or rectum, may be damaged during treatment.

The Nature of Cancer

• Prostate cancer can grow for a long time—even years—before it causes any symptoms. It is often not detected until it has reached an advanced stage.

• Cancerous cells can grow at several sites within the prostate and still not show up in the specific tissue samples collected for microscopic analysis.

• If cancer cells break out of the prostate, they can metastasize, or spread, to other organs and tissues in the body. It may not be possible to detect that spread until surgery is performed, at which time it may be too late for a cure.

Number of Treatments Available

In the early stages of prostate cancer, a man may be faced with a bewildering array of treatment options. Becoming educated about these choices is a challenge.

Lack of Scientific Evidence Proving Which Treatments Are Best

Naturally, you'd like to know with absolute certainty which treatments work best and pose the lowest risks. Studies that might provide these answers are still under way.

Differences of Opinion Among Experts

Even trained professionals may differ in their opinions about the best treatment program for you. People who seek a second opinion often hear the doctor say something completely different from what the first doctor said. Trying to reconcile these differences can be a challenge. Getting additional advice, whether from other physicians or from people with the disease, sometimes just adds to the confusion.

Differences Among Men with Prostate Cancer

A man in his early forties with an advanced form of prostate cancer is in a very different set of circumstances from a man in his eighties in an early stage of the disease. Similarly, a man who can't bear the thought that cancer is growing inside his body will demand a different treatment than will a man who is unwilling (or physically unable) to undergo a major operation that poses risks he finds unacceptable.

Physical and Psychological Impact of Treatment

Surgery or radiation can damage the urinary and reproductive organs, possibly leading to loss of urinary control and/or impotence. Hormone therapy, which may involve surgical removal of the testicles, can cause mood changes, hot flashes, and loss of interest in sex. At the very least, these problems disrupt a man's normal way of life. One man may feel the benefit of a longer, cancer-free life justifies these sacrifices. Another man may feel his self-esteem, his deepest sense of himself as a man, has been shattered. He may become depressed, lose interest in life, and withdraw from family and friends. As one woman remarked, "Prostate cancer is a disease that strikes men, but it affects the whole family."

REASONS TO HOPE

While there is a lot of confusion and controversy surrounding the diagnosis and treatment of prostate cancer, it is equally true that in recent years medicine has made tremendous strides forward.

For example, the advent of the prostate-specific antigen (PSA) blood test has made earlier detection possible, which in turn increases chances for a cure. PSA levels are also invaluable in monitoring the success of treatment, indicating when it is time to take additional steps.

New technology enhances our ability to evaluate what is going on inside the prostate and make more enlightened decisions based on what we find. Computerized tomography (CT), magnetic resonance imaging (MRI), and nuclear medicine scans can help us estimate whether the cancer has spread and if it has, to choose the safest and best therapy for that individual.

In the past decade, doctors have learned a great deal about both the anatomy of the prostate and the nature of prostate cancer. As a result of better understanding the arrangement of blood vessels, surgeons can now remove the prostate with minimal blood loss, thus avoiding the need for transfusions. A surgical technique developed at Johns Hopkins University makes it possible in some cases to preserve the nerves that facilitate erections. Improved biopsy tools and techniques have improved our ability to detect prostate cancer and determine how aggressive it is.

Refinements in treatment are also yielding results. Modern radiation therapy delivers more powerful doses more accurately. New hormonal therapies and drug combinations can better control the progress of the disease in those for whom a cure is not possible. Scientific advances continue pointing the way to potentially effective new approaches.

One of the most important strides forward has been the advent of support networks for men with prostate cancer. Groups such as Man to Man and US TOO provide the kinds of help that doctors can't carry in their little black bags: guidance, encouragement, and love. With the growing realization of the impact of prostate cancer on marriages and families, many of these support groups have expanded their mission by reaching out to loved ones. During group meetings, members share experiences, exchange ideas and information, and learn strategies for coping with their fears and concerns. As you will discover through the personal stories in this book, support groups can make a world of difference in the quality of life.

WHO SHOULD READ THIS BOOK

In these pages we hope to provide information for as wide an audience as possible, but our primary audience is men whose prostate cancer has just been diagnosed and who are trying to learn as much as possible. Such men benefit greatly by talking with others to learn about their experiences and by finding out what to expect. In our practice, we urge patients to join a support network, if possible, *before* making any treatment decisions. We've designed this book to serve as a "support group in print."

This book will also be useful for:

• Men who have not been diagnosed with prostate cancer but who are curious to learn more about their bodies and the disease.

• Men at high risk of prostate cancer, especially African-Americans and those with a family history of cancer who need to understand the importance of early detection.

• Wives, partners, or significant others of men with prostate cancer, especially those whose mates are dealing with impotence or incontinence and who wish to preserve or restore their sense of intimacy and closeness.

• Friends and family members who want to understand what their loved one is going through.

• Members of the caring professions, such as counselors, therapists, and clergy, who need to understand the issues that men with prostate cancer must deal with.

Our primary audience, however, remains the man with newly diagnosed prostate cancer, and it is to him that most of our remarks are addressed.

OVERVIEW OF THE BOOK

The first chapters provide basic facts about the prostate and about cancer. If you have already done some homework, or if you want others in your family to understand what is happening to you, these chapters provide a basic review of the subject.

Many men find out they have prostate cancer before they know they even *have* a prostate—let alone know what this mysterious gland does. As we explain in chapter 1, the better you understand your anatomy, the better informed you will be about the treatment options available to you.

In chapter 2, you'll find a brief discussion of cancer: how cells become cancerous, how cancer grows, and how it spreads. If you learn some important facts about how your illness evolves over time, you can develop a better sense of the choices that will confront you in the years to come.

Chapter 3 discusses what is known about the causes of prostate cancer, who is at risk, and what, if anything, can be done to prevent it. Chapter 4 describes the tests doctors use to detect the disease. In chapter 5, we explain the essential classifications of prostate cancer: the *grade* (how aggressive it is) and the *stage* (the extent of the cancer). You'll become as familiar with the numbers involved as many men are with their favorite baseball player's lifetime stats.

In chapter 6 we help you create a plan for dealing with prostate cancer. We talk about facing difficult emotional issues, assessing yourself, and determining the best treatment options for you. We also describe what to look for when choosing your doctors, offer tips on how to communicate with your caregivers, and explain the decisions you and your loved ones will have to make. You are faced with some tough issues. Not to beat around the bush, you'll have to confront your mortality by asking yourself, "How do I want to live so that the rest of my years will be the best they can possibly be?"

Chapters 7 through 12 explain the wide range of treatment options available, from simply monitoring early-stage disease to the most aggressive forms of treatment. Chapter 13 examines how those treatments are applied in cases of advanced or recurring prostate cancer.

We next outline practical strategies for dealing with two of the most significant long-term complications of treatment for prostate cancer. For many, incontinence poses the greatest threat to their ability to enjoy a full and active life. Chapter 14 describes the techniques available to help minimize the inconvenience and embarrassment that arise from loss of urinary control. Other men find the impact of treatment on their sexuality to be the most significant adverse effect. In chapter 15, you'll discover that the loss of erections due to prostate cancer treatment does not necessarily spell the end of your sex life. A number of options are available that can restore full sexual function. Men are often surprised to learn that, even without erections, they can continue to satisfy their partners—and even experience orgasm themselves.

Chapter 16 presents first-hand experiences of men and their partners who have benefited from participation in support groups and other networks. This chapter addresses an often-overlooked aspect of recovery from prostate cancer: the emotional and psychological needs of men and their families. Denial, anger, fear, stress, and depression are just a few of the "side effects" of cancer and its treatment. Typically, men in our society may not be aware that such feelings are gnawing at them. Instead, they may bottle up their emotions, refusing to acknowledge or talk about them. As a result they become more withdrawn emotionally and socially.

It doesn't have to be that way. Counseling can help couples preserve their sense of intimacy. Effective new medications can relieve depression and anxiety. But perhaps the most important form of help comes from the support groups—networks of friends and allies who are wrestling with similar challenges. Often the best coping strategies emerge from frank and open discussions among members of these groups. Merely being in the same room with these people, or reading their words here, can send a powerful message: *You are not alone.*

American Cancer Society
PROSTATE CANCER

Chapter 1

Where Is Your Prostate and What Does It Do?

When you first heard about prostate cancer, you probably had little or no idea where your prostate is or what it does. That is not surprising. Most of us take our bodies for granted, and—as long as the prostate is working properly—there is little need to think much about this small internal organ. As you know by now, though, if something does go wrong with the prostate, the consequences can be enormous.

In this chapter, we describe the prostate's structure and function. Words in *italic* type are medical terms describing the different parts and functions of the prostate, the male reproductive system, and the urinary tract. We try to avoid using too much technical jargon, but we believe that if you know the basic terminology and understand how your body works, you will have a better understanding of what's happening to you right now and also a better grasp of the treatment options you discuss with your physician.

Don't worry if you find this information a little overwhelming at first. Some of it may make more sense after you have read the section on treatment options. And you may want to review specific parts of this chapter later, to place the information in a more meaningful context. For easy reference, we have included a glossary at the back of the book.

Now, down to the basics.

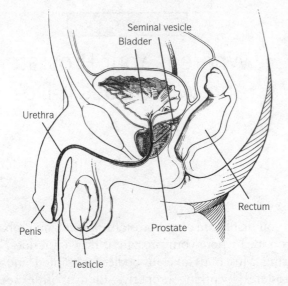

Figure 1.1: Male anatomy, showing location of the prostate.

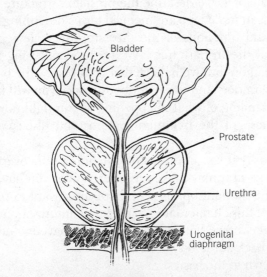

Figure 1.2: The prostate, indicating position of the urethra.

A BIOLOGIST'S DISCOVERY

A decade ago, Jim Mullen and his wife, Marian, were vacationing in South Carolina. Their trip was being spoiled, however, because Jim had to get up many times each night to go to the bathroom. Neither of them was getting much sleep, and they were unable to enjoy the sun, surf, and scenery. As is so often the way with wives, Marian insisted that Jim see a doctor, even though they were hundreds of miles from home. The doctor, after poking around with his finger, told Jim he suspected prostate cancer.

As Jim recalled later, he was puzzled by what the doctor told him. "I didn't even know what the prostate was. I'd never heard the word before." The fact that he was a trained professional biologist was no help. "I had been doing biological research for Du Pont for years, so I must have come across a reference to the prostate at one time or another. But somehow it just never sank in."

In the years to come, however, Jim learned a lot about the prostate. What's more, he has shared his findings with thousands of others. As the founder of Man to Man, a support group for survivors of prostate cancer, Jim has converted his former ignorance about the prostate into a life-saving nationwide network.

A QUICK ANATOMY LESSON

The prostate—a sex gland found only in men—is located inside the lower abdomen at the base of the penis, just below the bladder and in front of the rectum (Fig. 1.1). Normally the prostate is about an inch and a half in diameter—roughly the size of a golf ball. The *apex* (the end farthest from the bladder) is somewhat elongated, giving the prostate the shape of a small upside-down pear. Your doctor can feel some parts of the prostate during a *digital rectal examination* (DRE), when he inserts a gloved finger into your rectum.

The prostate wraps completely around the *urethra*, the tube that empties urine from the bladder through the penis (Fig. 1.2). The

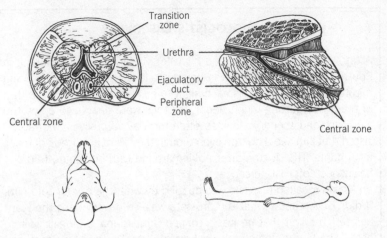

Figure 1.3: Side and top views of the prostate.

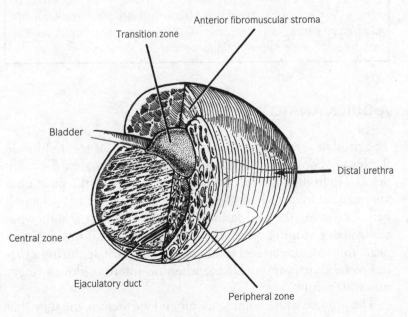

Figure 1.4: Zones of the prostate.

WHAT'S IN A WORD?

It is not unusual for people to mix up the words *prostrate* and *prostate*. *Prostrate*—with a *tr*—comes from a Latin word meaning "to throw down." Used as a verb, it means to lie flat or prone, or to kneel or bow down in humility or adoration. As an adjective, it describes someone who is lying in that position.

Prostate (only one "r") derives from Greek *pro* ("before") and *status* ("standing"), and it refers to the fact that the prostate gland "stands before" the bladder.

One of our patients says he keeps the two words straight by remembering the phrase, "You are prone to be prostrate when they examine your prostate!"

prostate is also connected to the male reproductive organs. The *vasa deferentia* (two tubes that carry sperm from the testicles into the urethra; the singular form—often used to refer to both structures—is *vas deferens*) and the *seminal vesicles* (two clusters of little sacs that contribute fluid to your semen) all drain into the prostate.

THE PURPOSE OF THE PROSTATE

The prostate gland manufactures *prostatic fluid,* which forms part of your *semen,* the milky liquid that you ejaculate during orgasm. In addition to prostatic fluid, semen contains fluid from the seminal vesicles and sperm from the testicles; the sperm make up less than 1 percent of semen. One specific function of prostatic fluid is to regulate the acidity of semen. Prostatic fluid is highly alkaline, which protects sperm as it travels through the acid environment of the female reproductive tract.

Besides producing prostatic fluid, the prostate acts as a valve that allows sperm and urine to flow in the right direction: out of the body through the urethra. It also functions as a pump. When you have an orgasm, the prostate's muscular tissue contracts, forcing semen into the urethra. A ring of muscles (the bladder neck) surrounding the urethra near the base of the prostate clamps down to prevent semen from flowing into the bladder during ejaculation.

The prostate is part of your urinary and reproductive systems (also known as the *urogenital system*), but it is not really a vital organ. In other words, it is similar to the gallbladder—you can live without it, although most men, given the option, prefer to live *with* it.

STRUCTURE OF THE PROSTATE

It may be small, but the prostate is a complicated organ (Figs. 1.3 and 1.4). It contains two main kinds of tissue: the *smooth muscle* and hundreds of tiny, spongy *glands*. Because it has these two different kinds of tissue, the prostate is sometimes described as a *musculoglandular* structure.

Outer Coat

Most of the prostate is surrounded by a thin, fibrous membrane sometimes called the *capsule*. If cancerous cells manage to escape from the prostate through this outer layer, they can circulate to other tissues of the body. From that point on, prostate cancer is more difficult to cure and sometimes can only be controlled. Surgery for prostate cancer involves removing both the outer layer and the internal glandular tissue. Other kinds of surgery—for example, to treat certain forms of noncancerous enlargement of the prostate—treat only the inner part of the gland.

Zones of the Prostate

The prostate is divided into three zones (refer back to Figs. 1.3 and 1.4). The largest is the *peripheral zone*, which contains about 70 percent of the prostate's glandular tissue. Most prostate cancer

WHAT IS A GLAND?

Glands are groups of cells whose purpose is to make and release chemical products for use by other parts of the body. *Endocrine glands,* such as the adrenals and the pituitary, make substances such as hormones or enzymes that act on various internal organs. *Exocrine glands,* including the sweat and salivary glands, release substances either onto the skin or into hollow body structures, such as the mouth or digestive tract.

Although it is often described as a gland, the prostate is actually a collection of innumerable small glandular units, or prostatic *acini* (pronounced AH-sin-eye), that are grouped into one organ. These acini produce the prostatic fluid that makes up about 30 to 50 percent of semen.

begins in the peripheral zone. This is the only tissue a doctor can feel by digital rectal examination and is the tissue most often sampled during a needle biopsy.

The rest of the prostate's glandular tissues are found in the smaller *central* and *transition zones.* The transition zone completely surrounds the urethra and is usually the smallest of the three zones. Some prostate cancers, and virtually all cases of BPH (benign prostatic hyperplasia, a noncancerous enlargement of the prostate), begin in this tissue. Prostate cancer rarely begins in the central zone, which is at the base of the prostate, nearest the bladder.

The other major region of the prostate is the *anterior tissue,* which is mostly made up of smooth muscle and is not usually involved in prostatic disease.

NEARBY STRUCTURES

The prostate lies in close proximity to other tissues and organs, and its function is intimately connected with theirs. As previously mentioned, the urethra passes through the middle of the prostate, as do the ejaculatory ducts from the seminal vesicles. Tucked right under the bladder, the prostate lies directly in front of the rectum. All these structures are kept alive and nourished by a delicate and complex network of nerves and blood vessels. Nerves that run alongside the prostate, contained within the neurovascular bundles, are responsible for making the penis become hard during an erection. As you'll learn in subsequent chapters, the presence of all these tissues complicates treatment choices enormously, because therapies that are focused on one area may have indirect, unwanted effects on other areas. Removing the erectile nerves, for example, means naturally occurring erections are no longer possible.

HORMONES: THE CHEMICAL MESSENGERS THAT MAKE THE PROSTATE GROW

In childhood, the prostate is only about the size of a pea. During puberty, the body begins producing large amounts of male hormones, or *androgens,* which cause the prostate to grow rapidly to its adult size and shape.

The most important form of androgen is *testosterone.* Most testosterone—about 95 percent—is produced by the testicles. Triggering prostate growth is just one function of androgens. These powerful chemicals also control all aspects of the body change known as *virilization:* growth of the scrotum, testicles, and penis; development of body hair; deepening of the voice; and increase in muscle bulk, especially in the chest and shoulders. Androgens also cause the prostate to begin manufacturing prostatic fluid.

Once your prostate reaches normal adult size, it generally stops growing until you reach middle age. At that point it often starts to enlarge even more, probably because of the complex hormonal changes associated with aging. Over time, an enlarged prostate may start to squeeze the urethra, affecting the ability to

WHAT DO ANDROGENS DO?

Besides stimulating the development of certain sexual characteristics, androgens such as testosterone are involved in a number of physical and mental events in the body. Some of the effects of androgens are controversial, especially their role in triggering male aggression and hostility. Still, the consequences of having too much or too little of these essential hormones have been well defined.

Androgen excess in prepubertal males:
  • Premature sexual development
  • Shorter average height

Androgen excess in women:
  • Increased body and facial hair
  • Deepening of voice
  • Enlargement of clitoris
  • Absence of menstruation

Androgen deficiency (men only):
  • Decreased body and facial hair
  • High-pitched voice
  • Underdeveloped genitals
  • Lack of muscle development
  • Reduced sex drive

urinate. This gradual increase in size of the prostate leads to the condition called *benign prostatic hyperplasia*, or *BPH*. As the word *benign* indicates, BPH is rarely a threat to health, but it can cause uncomfortable and even severe symptoms.

The action of testosterone on the prostate is part of a complex chain of biochemical events. First, a tiny gland in the brain, the *hypothalamus*, pumps out *luteinizing hormone–releasing hormone (LHRH)*. The LHRH travels to the nearby pituitary gland and signals the pituitary to secrete hormones known as *go-*

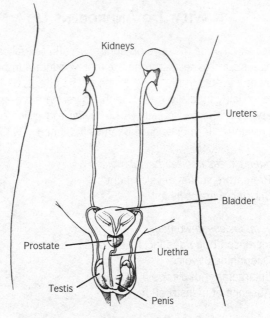

Figure 1.5: Male urinary system.

nadotropins. (The word basically means "chemicals that turn on the gonads.") One of these gonadotropins is *luteinizing hormone* (*LH*). LH circulates to the testicles, which respond by releasing testosterone into the blood stream.

Once in circulation, some of the testosterone travels to the prostate, where it is absorbed by individual prostate cells. Inside the cell, an enzyme (called *5-alpha reductase*) converts the testosterone into *dihydrotestosterone*, or *DHT*. The DHT then migrates to the cell's nucleus, rolls up its sleeves, and goes to work.

In addition to the androgens produced by the testicles, some androgens are produced by the adrenal glands in both men and women. In response to hormonal signals from the hypothalamus, the pituitary gland secretes a substance called *ACTH* (short for *adrenocorticotropic hormone*). This hormone travels to the adrenal glands and stimulates them to produce adrenal androgens, which are not as powerful as the androgens produced by the testicles. For example, they don't usually cause virilization unless abnormally large amounts are produced.

Besides driving prostate growth, androgens also fuel the growth of prostate cancer cells, the way gasoline fuels a fire. That's why, as we'll explain in chapter 10, one option for some men with prostate cancer is hormone therapy, which works by affecting one or more links in the chain of hormonal events. By disrupting the production and distribution of hormones, these treatments may stop, or at least slow down, the progress of prostate disease.

THE PROSTATE'S ROLE IN URINATION

Because of the way the prostate surrounds the urethra, prostate diseases can have a major impact on urination. To understand the problem, here's a quick guided tour of the male urinary system (Fig. 1.5).

Kidneys

The urinary tract begins with the *kidneys*, two bean-shaped organs roughly the size of your fists that lie on either side of the spine at the bottom of the rib cage. The kidneys filter out toxic wastes, excess water, and salts from the blood. At the same time, they salvage useful materials and recycle them into the bloodstream.

Ureters

In the average man, the kidneys produce about two quarts of urine a day. The urine drains into two muscular tubes called the *ureters*, which squeeze the urine out of the kidneys, pushing it down into the *bladder*. The ureters pass through the wall of the bladder, forming a one-way-valve mechanism that allows urine to flow into the bladder but does not allow it to flow back up into the kidneys.

Bladder

The bladder is basically a muscular reservoir for urine. As it fills, the bladder expands, and as it empties, it contracts. Most of the time we can choose when we want to eliminate urine. Problems with the muscle in the bladder or other urinary structures, however, can reduce our ability to regulate urination. As a result, urine can dribble or leak out. This condition is known as *incontinence*. As previously mentioned, treatments for prostate cancer can seriously damage urinary control, resulting in incontinence.

Urethra

Urine is propelled from the bladder into the urethra. This tube, about eight inches long, tunnels through the prostate at an angle, then travels down through the penis. If the prostate becomes enlarged—whether through cancerous growth or from a benign condition—the urethra may be constricted or narrowed, preventing urine from flowing properly.

THE PROSTATE AND SEXUAL FUNCTION

Besides being part of the urinary tract, the prostate forms part of the male reproductive system, which also includes the testicles, the epididymis, the vasa deferentia, the seminal vesicles, the ejaculatory ducts, and the penis (all described below). Problems in the prostate or any of these other areas can impair fertility. They can also interfere with the ability to have an erection or to experience orgasm and ejaculation.

When considering the role of the prostate in sexual function, it's important to keep a few key concepts straight:

• *Fertility* means the ability to reproduce—that is, to manufacture and deliver healthy sperm capable of reaching and fertilizing an egg from a woman's body.

• *Ejaculation* is the release of semen during orgasm.

• *Potency* means the ability to have and maintain an erection capable of penetrating the vagina and sustaining sexual intercourse.

Medically speaking, *potency* is not the same as the ability to father a child.

Another distinction: ejaculation is not the same as orgasm. You can have an orgasm without expelling any fluid; this is known as a *dry orgasm.*

It should also be pointed out that *sperm* and *semen* are not synonyms. Ejaculate contains several different fluids. Semen from men who have had vasectomies does not contain sperm, but it does contain seminal fluid and prostatic fluid.

One final note, and this can't be stressed enough: *Even if you can't get an erection, you can still have an orgasm.* The nerves involved are completely different. Usually the orgasmic nerves are not affected by treatment for prostate cancer. There is no denying that cancer treatment can have a serious impact on sexual function. But as you'll learn in chapter 15, it can still be possible to enjoy a mutually satisfying sexual relationship with your partner if you are willing to communicate openly about your needs and work together to discover new forms of intimacy.

Testicles

The testicles, which get their blood supply from a vessel known as the testicular artery in the spermatic cord, are responsible for the production of sperm. Immature sperm are manufactured in hundreds of tiny compartments, or tubules, within the testicle. Then they migrate by the millions to the epididymis, where they mature.

The testicles are also the main (but not the only) source of testosterone, which, as you know, can stimulate tumor growth. In cases of prostate disease, strategies to eliminate testosterone include the use of drugs that block its production or the surgical removal of the testicles (also known as *orchiectomy* or *castration*).

Epididymis

Each testicle has one of these structures, which "incubate" sperm produced by the testicles until they mature. During orgasm, the muscles around the epididymis contract with great force, propelling the mature sperm into the *vas deferens*.

Vas Deferens

There are two *vasa deferentia* (plural), thick, muscular tubes, one running from each testicle to the prostate. A vas deferens has only one function: to pump sperm to the part of the urethra located within the prostate. Anatomically speaking, this is a relatively long distance — a total of about eighteen inches. At the base of the prostate, each vas deferens joins the duct of a seminal vesicle at the upper back (posterior) of the prostate, where it forms the *ejaculatory duct*. The vasa deferentia are the tubes that are cut and tied off in a *vasectomy*, the surgical procedure some men choose as a means of birth control.

Ejaculatory Duct

The ejaculatory duct passes into the prostate through the central zone and connects with the urethra at an anatomic juncture called the *verumontanum*.

Seminal Vesicles

The two *seminal vesicles* join with the vasa deferentia just before they enter the prostate. These glandular organs, which look like two-inch-long clusters of tiny grapes, rest on top of either side of the prostate. They produce a sticky secretion that helps maintain the proper consistency of semen.

Penis

The penis is a complex structure made up of nerves, smooth muscle, and blood vessels. It becomes erect thanks to a well-engineered hydraulic system. Under normal conditions, sexual stimulation causes the nerves in the penis to instruct the arteries to expand and to retain extra blood. The nerves then signal the veins to constrict so that the blood comes in but cannot flow out as quickly. As the blood fills up the three hollow, spongy tissue structures in the penis—the two *corpora cavernosa* and the *corpus spongiosum*—erection occurs.

Many of the nerves that control erection run along either side of the prostate. If cancer cells penetrate the prostate and enter the nerves on one or both sides, the nerves must be removed during surgery. This can lead to impotence, or the inability to have an erection. Again, bear in mind that *impotence does not mean you can no longer have sex*. It may mean you cannot achieve penetration on your own, but as you'll learn in chapter 15, there are many options available to help you.

Chapter 2

What Is Cancer?

Cancer: one of the most dreaded words in human language. It packs a tremendous emotional punch, conjuring images of pain, suffering, debilitation, and death.

Cancer is not a single disease, but a group of diseases. All cancers share one trait in common: They are composed of cells that exhibit uncontrolled growth and division. Despite this similarity, you must understand this crucial point: *Every case of cancer is different.* It is not possible to compare what happened during Aunt Betty's breast cancer to Uncle Charlie's colon cancer, or to your own prostate cancer. These cancers each affect a different part of the body; each is treated differently and each has a different prognosis.

Strange as it may sound, prostate cancer can be one of the "better" cancers to get, because it is both slow-growing and treatable. And if it is detected early enough, there is an excellent chance for a cure. In the next chapter, we discuss the simple blood test (PSA) that can assist with early diagnosis and monitoring of prostate cancer. Even more encouraging, there are a number of treatments that can suppress the disease and keep it from becoming life threatening. Over 90 percent of men with early-stage prostate cancer will live at *least* another five years; many will live much longer. What's more, prospects are good even when the tumor is not detected in its earliest stages. Studies find that about half of men whose prostate cancer has spread outside the gland will survive for five years *or longer.*

The bottom line: Prostate cancer is by no means a death sentence. Most men with prostate cancer can look forward to enjoying healthy, productive lives for many years to come.

TYPES OF CANCER

The four major types of cancer are classified according to the type of tissue in which the cancers begin.

• *Carcinoma* is a solid tumor that develops in the epithelial tissues that surround all parts of the body, including the internal organs. Carcinoma is the most common type of cancer and includes cancers of the prostate, breast, lung, colon, intestine, and skin.

• *Sarcoma* develops in bone or connective tissue.

• *Lymphoma* arises in the lymph system, usually in the lymph nodes.

• *Leukemia* begins in the blood system, usually in bone marrow where blood cells are formed.

Remember, your prostate cancer is not the same as anyone else's. Resist the temptation to compare what's happening to you with what happened to your fishing buddy or that guy in the next office. Everything about your case is unique, from the location of the tumor within the prostate to the emotional and psychological resources you bring to bear on the problem.

Understanding the general nature of cancer—how it affects cells, how it grows, how it spreads—will help you grasp the specific characteristics of prostate cancer. It will also give you insight into your treatment options and help you understand how prostate cancer is very different from other conditions that affect the prostate.

NORMAL CELLS

There are four major types of cancer and hundreds of different subtypes. To understand what is abnormal about cancer cells, let's take a moment first to discuss what a normal cell is.

Cells are the basic units that make up all tissues. Your body is made up of billions of cells. There are many different types of cells with different functions throughout the body, but they all act together to carry out the countless complex tasks of keeping you alive. Each of the cells of the prostate has a specialized function. Most are glandular cells, which produce prostatic secretions. A smaller proportion are cells that make up the smooth muscles, which propel prostatic secretions and seminal fluid into the urethra.

The growth and behavior of a cell are controlled by its genetic material, or *DNA*, which is stored inside the nucleus of the cell. The DNA is made up of many genes, each of which contain coded instructions telling the cell what to do: when to produce certain proteins, how to repair DNA damage, when to divide, and even when to die.

As old cells die, they are continually replaced with healthy new cells (except in the heart and brain, where cells are not replaced). In most cases, the adult body makes just enough new cells to replace those that have died, a process called *cellular replication*.

ABNORMAL CELLS

If a cell contains damaged genes, the cell may begin to behave abnormally. One possible result is uncontrolled cell division, which is cancer.

Researchers have found at least three mechanisms that affect the growth of cancerous cells. We'll briefly discuss each of these.

Receptor Abnormalities

The surface membranes of cells are normally studded with molecules called *receptors*. Receptors have a precise shape and they function like little "receiving docks." If a molecule with just the right shape, such as a hormone molecule, docks to the receptor, a message is sent to the nucleus of the cell, causing the DNA to perform a preprogrammed task. In some cancers, though, these cell receptors are abnormal in some way: There may be too many of them, they may be oversensitive to stimulation, they may respond to wrong-shaped proteins, or they may simply send the wrong message back to the nucleus. Whatever the cause, the effect is that the nuclear DNA reacts by doing what it thinks it is being told to do: Multiply, multiply, multiply.

Oncogenes

All dividing cells have genes (known as *proto-oncogenes*) whose role is to orchestrate normal replication. Usually these proto-oncogenes are kept under control. In some cancers, however, proto-oncogenes escape normal control mechanisms and start to drive the replication process relentlessly. When this happens, the proto-oncogene has become an *oncogene*, and the cell multiplies out of control until it becomes a cancer.

Tumor Suppressor Genes

Normal cells abide by the instructions contained in certain genes called *tumor suppressor genes*. These genes prevent a cell from misbehaving: replicating at the wrong time, wandering away from "home" without permission, or any other action that could threaten the health of the body. As a safeguard, every cell starts out with two identical copies of these genetic "rule books," with the second set acting as a backup. In cancer, however, the "text" of the rule book is garbled. In some instances, the DNA is damaged so badly that it cannot be repaired. Losing one set of suppressor genes isn't a disaster, because the cell is still controlled by the remaining normal set. However, if *both* sets are damaged or destroyed, the cell replicates endlessly. What's more, there may be nothing to stop these cells from migrating—*metastasizing*—to other parts of the body.

When cells become cancerous, they no longer perform their specialized functions. Instead, they essentially become parasites, consuming the energy and nutrients that the body's normal cells

---

MALIGNANT AND BENIGN TUMORS

Cancers are often referred to as *malignant tumors* or *malignant neoplasms*. They are not, however, the only type of abnormal growth that occurs in the body. There are also numerous noncancerous, *benign* tumors or neoplasms, such as warts and polyps.

Cancers differ from benign tumors in two essential ways: The first is that as cancers grow, they infiltrate surrounding tissues.

The second way that cancers differ from benign tumors is that they can *metastasize*—that is, cells from the original cancer (the *primary tumor*) may spread to other parts of the body through the blood vessels or the lymph system. These traveling cells can form new tumors that grow independently of the primary tumor.

---

need to thrive. They also become so numerous that they literally crowd out healthy cells.

The abnormal cells usually show a lack of *differentiation*—that is, they are no longer able to perform the specialized function of the parent cell. Seen under a microscope, cancer cells look jumbled and disordered, in stark contrast to the relative uniformity and order of normal cells.

HOW MALIGNANCY DEVELOPS

A tumor is a swelling or a growth. A cancerous tumor is a collection of cells that often infiltrates other tissue as it grows and metastasizes to other parts of the body.

Despite popular belief, cancer cells do not always divide *faster* than normal cells. Rather, cancerous tumors get bigger because in any given population of cancer cells, more of them are actively dividing at any one time, relentlessly causing the tumor to increase in size. Some cancer cells even become "immortal"—they no longer have the genetic instructions that program them to self-destruct.

As a colony of malignant cells expands, it invades and crowds out the normal tissue surrounding it. The growing tumor can destroy healthy tissue directly by compressing it, but it can also cause damage indirectly, by infiltrating nearby tissues or growing through open spaces in the body (for example, the abdominal cavity). As the cancer spreads, internal passageways are blocked off and the surrounding normal tissues are robbed of the nutrients they need to thrive.

HOW CANCER SPREADS

Malignant tumors—those that are capable of endangering health and life—are generally divided into three categories:

• *Localized* tumors remain within the boundaries of the tissues where they began.

• *Regional* tumors have invaded neighboring tissues.

• *Metastasized* tumors have spread to other parts of the body.

Tumors metastasize when one or more cancer cells break away from the primary tumor. If these cells make their way into the bloodstream or the lymphatic system, they can then circulate to other tissues and organs, where they can lodge and cause new colonies of cancer cells to grow.

The most frequent sites for *metastasis* are the liver, lungs, and bones. When prostate cancer spreads, its first destination is usually the nearby lymph nodes in the lower abdomen. This is why many men with prostate cancer undergo a lymph node dissection prior to radical prostatectomy or curative radiation therapy: The physicians want to study the nodes to see if the cancer has already escaped from the prostate.

Cancer is always identified by the site of the original or *primary* tumor, even when it spreads to another part of the body. If it arises in the prostate, then it is called prostate cancer. If it metastasizes to bone, it is called metastatic prostate cancer, not bone cancer. The distinction is important, because it determines the type of treatment possible.

RATE OF CANCER GROWTH

Different cancers grow at different speeds. In discussing growth, your doctor will usually refer to a tumor's *doubling rate*, which means the time it takes for the number of cells in the tumor to increase by 100 percent. Some tumors, such as certain lung cancers, double very rapidly. Others grow relatively slowly, and years may pass before the cancer doubles enough times to cause any symptoms. Fortunately, most prostate cancer is slow growing, with doubling rates measured in years.

The potential for a tumor to spread to other tissues is related to three factors:

One factor is its size or volume. The larger the tumor is, the more likely it is to grow into neighboring tissues.

The second factor is the degree of cell *differentiation*—that is, the extent to which the cancerous cells resemble the normal cells from which they arose. Well-differentiated cancer cells, ones that still resemble the original cells, are less likely to spread. Poorly differentiated cells tend to be more virulent.

The third factor that determines a tumor's invasiveness is the number of small blood vessels that nourish it, what scientists call *microvessel density*. Recent studies show that, compared to other cancers, prostate cancer needs a relatively high microvessel density in order to grow and metastasize.

PROSTATE CANCER

Prostate cancer begins when something triggers abnormal growth of cells in the prostate. Unfortunately, we don't yet know just what that something is. In chapter 3, we talk more about the factors that seem to increase a man's risk of getting prostate cancer. At highest risk in this country are older men and African-Americans, but such factors as heredity, environment, and hormones also can play a role.

Cancerous growth can start at a number of different sites within the prostate. The most common site of origin is the *peripheral zone*, the main glandular section of the prostate. Because this type of prostate cancer arises from glandular cells, it is called an *adenocarcinoma*. The prefix *adeno-* means "pertaining to a gland," and *carcinoma* means a cancer that develops in *epithelial* cells (cells surrounding an organ or body tissue, such as a gland).

More than 99 percent of prostate cancers are adenocarcinomas. Cancer rarely begins in the other (nonglandular) tissues of the prostate. All the more unusual forms of prostate cancer together account for less than 1 percent of all cases. These tumors include *sarcomas, squamous cell carcinomas, urothelial carcinomas, carcinosarcomas,* and *lymphomas*. Because they are so uncommon, a detailed discussion of these types of prostate cancer is beyond the scope of this book.

A WORD ABOUT PROSTATIC INTRAEPITHELIAL NEOPLASIA (PIN)

You may hear your doctor describe abnormal cells as *precancerous* or *dysplastic*, or say that you have *PIN*. These terms indicate something wrong with the cells' size, shape, or the rate at which they multiply. PIN is a condition that *may* lead to the development of the most common type of prostate cancer—that is, prostatic adenocarcinoma. In PIN, there are changes in the microscopic appearance of prostatic epithelial cells. Most urologists and pathologists believe that these mutations represent a precursor of cancer; that is, the earliest stage of cellular changes that can eventually develop into prostate cancer. As with other prostate conditions, the incidence of PIN is related to age: The older you are, the more likely you are to have it. But PIN appears at a much younger age — usually at least ten or twenty years before prostate cancer develops. If, during a routine checkup, a man's digital rectal examination is negative but a PSA test is positive, his doctor may recommend a biopsy.

If PIN is then found, the condition is classified as either *low grade* or *high grade*. Low grade PIN is no cause for alarm, and some pathologists don't even report this finding. High grade PIN, however, is a call to action. Repeat biopsies and PSA tests should be done regularly to make sure there is no trace of prostate cancer. Right now, there is no accepted treatment for PIN, but studies are being done to see if any drug treatments, including those used for BPH, might reverse PIN.

WHERE PROSTATE TUMORS BEGIN

Most tumors begin at the outer back part of the prostate, in the epithelial cells of the peripheral zone. Since the tumor starts so far from the urethra, a long time can elapse before growth interferes with the flow of urine and causes symptoms. As the tumor grows, however, the prostate gland enlarges and becomes hardened and lumpy, or *nodular*. Eventually, the tumor can start to obstruct the urethra, but this is a late development that usually indicates an advanced cancer.

Even if the tumor does not produce symptoms, an early diagnosis of prostate cancer is possible. Because of a fortunate feature of male anatomical design, the posterior surface of the prostate is very close to the rectum. As a result, many prostate cancers can be felt during a DRE. And even before it can be felt, as the tumor develops, its cancerous cells begin to produce higher levels of a substance called *prostate-specific antigen*, or PSA. Like DRE, PSA is an extremely useful tool for detecting prostate cancer, even in its earliest stages. Both of these screening tests are discussed in detail in chapter 4.

HOW PROSTATE CANCER GROWS

It is possible to have a tumor in your prostate for years before you even know it is there. Prostate cancer is so slow growing that many men die *with* prostate cancer, not *because* of it. Even if cancer is diagnosed at a late stage, there are a number of treatments that may suppress its growth and relieve many of its symptoms.

Some prostate cancers can be very aggressive, however. It is impossible to predict with certainty how active the specific disease in any one person will be. Sometimes the tumor grows so slowly that it never spreads beyond the prostate. If it does, though, the cancer can spread to many other parts of the body, first by invading the nearby seminal vesicles and then metastasizing via the blood and lymph vessels. The most common places for metastatic prostate cancer to take hold are the lymph nodes and the bones in the pelvis and lower spine. However, since the blood circulation and lymph system nourish the entire body, new tumors may take root practically anywhere, including other bones such as the ribs or skull, or other internal organs such as the liver or lungs.

SYMPTOMS OF PROSTATE CANCER

Many people are familiar with the American Cancer Society's seven warning signals of cancer. Unfortunately, that list doesn't often apply to prostate cancer, which is usually *asymptomatic*— that is, it may progress without any warning signals at all. In most cases today, the diagnosis of prostate cancer is made either as the result of a routine screening or unexpectedly as the result of some other test or procedure.

Eventually, as the tumor develops, it may press on the urethra and cause urinary symptoms, which can be described as either *irritative* or *obstructive* (see box, p. 29). In addition to the urinary symptoms, prostate cancer can also result in more generalized symptoms, including pain in the lower back or pelvic area.

You may have prostate cancer without having any of these symptoms. By the same token, having these symptoms does not necessarily mean that you *do* have prostate cancer. These symptoms are *nonspecific*, which means they can be found in other conditions. In making a diagnosis, your doctor will differentiate among the various possibilities, described in more detail in the next section.

COMPARING CANCERS

Because cancer can affect cells in so many different ways, it is impossible to predict the outcome of cancer in one person based on the experience of another. Moreover, the severity of symptoms is not necessarily related to the severity of the disease. You cannot assume that your cancer is worse than someone else's because you have symptoms and he does not, or because your symptoms seem worse than his.

The unique nature of each individual case of prostate cancer is often the source of enormous confusion. You might read an article in which an expert states that Tumor X has a survival rate of Y years. But this information tells you only what the *average* is for everyone who is diagnosed with that particular type of malignancy, using the treatments available at the time that study was done. It does *not* tell you about how you or any other individual will respond to treatment, or how *you* will fare in the coming years.

The fact that your prostate cancer is not like anyone else's can result in tremendous frustration when it comes time to make choices about therapy. It means you cannot usually base your decision on what happened to someone else. That person's age, or general state of health, or the precise location of the tumor in his prostate, his PSA level—even the part of the country where he makes his home—can affect the outcome. With so many factors involved, an absolutely precise, clear, and consistent way to predict the results of various therapies simply does not exist.

Ironically, though, this diversity is also a source of enormous hope.

SIGNS AND SYMPTOMS OF PROSTATE CANCER

In the earliest stages, most cases of prostate cancer do not cause *any* symptoms. When symptoms do occur, they may include one or more of the following. However, many of these signs and symptoms are also encountered with nonmalignant prostatic diseases, such as BPH and prostatitis.

Urinary Signs and Symptoms
- Irritative
    - Urgent need to urinate (*urgency*)
    - Frequent urination (*frequency*)
    - Urination at night (*nocturia*)
    - Painful urination (*dysuria*)
    - Urinary *incontinence* due to urgency
- Obstructive
    - Difficulty getting the stream started (*hesitancy*)
    - Weak or interrupted urinary stream
    - Feeling that bladder is full after urination (*incomplete emptying*)
    - Urinary incontinence due to overflow from a distended bladder

Other Signs and Symptoms
- Pain in lower back or pelvic area
- Loss of appetite
- Weight loss

Why?

Because a treatment that does not work for one person might be just right for you.

NONCANCEROUS CONDITIONS OF THE PROSTATE

Not every abnormal condition of the prostate is cancer. Two conditions often confused with prostate cancer—benign prostatic hyperplasia and prostatitis—have no relationship to prostate cancer at all. In addition, having either of these conditions does not increase a man's risk of developing prostate cancer.

Benign Prostatic Hyperplasia (BPH)

Hyperplasia, or enlargement, of the prostate is one of the most common disorders affecting middle-aged and older men. More than half of men over the age of sixty have some degree of BPH.

BPH typically affects the *transition zone* of the prostate—a distinct collection of prostatic glands next to the urethral channel, where prostate cancer rarely develops. When a man reaches his thirties or forties, the tissues in the transition zone typically begin to enlarge as the prostate glands and the tissues supporting them begin to proliferate. We simply don't know why this proliferation, or hyperplasia, occurs. In some cases, this enlargement obstructs the flow of urine through the urethra.

The urinary symptoms of BPH may resemble those experienced by some men with prostate cancer. It can be difficult to start urinating, the stream may be weak, and the bladder may not feel completely empty. The symptoms of BPH usually develop gradually. If similar symptoms are caused by cancer, they tend to worsen more rapidly—over the course of months instead of years.

If urinary symptoms of BPH are bothersome, they can often be relieved by either medication or surgery. One medication used for BPH (finasteride, sold under the trade name of Proscar), is currently being studied to see if it might also prevent the development of prostate cancer. There are also surgical treatments, such as *transurethral resection of the prostate* (TURP), that are sometimes used both for BPH and in the management of prostate cancer.

Although BPH and prostate cancer may cause similar urinary symptoms, *having BPH does not increase a man's risk for prostate cancer*. Nevertheless, men with BPH need to be screened regularly for prostate cancer, because the two conditions can exist together.

Prostatitis

Prostatitis is a general term used for conditions that result in inflammation of the prostate gland. Usual symptoms include painful or burning urination and the need to void frequently; less common symptoms include fever, discharge from the penis, blood in the urine, and pain in the lower back or lower abdomen.

Acute prostatitis and *chronic bacterial prostatitis* are the result of infection by bacteria; the cause of *nonbacterial prostatitis* is unknown. A fourth condition, *prostatodynia*, has the same symptoms as prostatitis but is usually caused by muscle spasms in structures that are near the prostate, rather than in the prostate itself.

Symptoms can develop suddenly and dramatically in acute bacterial prostatitis; they are generally milder in chronic disease. The acute form usually responds well to treatment with antibiotic drugs, but chronic bacterial prostatitis can take weeks or months to clear up and commonly recurs.

Antibiotics are useless against nonbacterial prostatitis, which is the most common form of prostatitis; they also are ineffective in prostatodynia. Other treatments, including anti-inflammatory drugs, sitz baths, and alpha-blockers (also used in BPH to relax compression of the urethra) may help relieve the symptoms of prostatitis when antibiotics do not work.

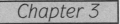

Why Did I Get Prostate Cancer?

A man's first reaction to the news that he has prostate cancer is usually shock, followed by denial and anger. Then he may start to wonder, *Why me?* The fact is, if you are a man and you live long enough, there is a good chance that you will eventually develop prostate cancer. Autopsy studies show that although only about 3 percent of men over age fifty die from prostate cancer, more than 50 percent have the disease at the time of death, and many of these cases were diagnosed only at autopsy. Today, even though prostate cancer is being diagnosed with increasing frequency, the odds that it will prove fatal are declining because of earlier detection and better treatment.

No one really knows why certain men get prostate cancer, but there are plenty of theories. Some previously suspected culprits, such as having too much or too little sex, have been discredited. Other factors—age, genetic heritage, and certain environmental elements—do play some role, but we do not understand just what that role is. Keep in mind that risk factors are simply conditions that are *associated* with an increased likelihood of disease. They cannot predict which individuals within even a high-risk group will develop the disease.

EXTENT OF THE PROBLEM

The causes of prostate cancer may be unknown, but its impact is clear. An estimated one out of every ten men in the United States will receive a diagnosis of prostate cancer before he reaches the age of eighty-five. *(Note: Statistics in this section apply only to men in the United States; as we'll explain later, the numbers vary among different ethnic groups and in different parts of the world.)*

The statistics are particularly sobering when you consider that the *incidence*, or number of newly diagnosed cases, is on the rise. In 1993, 164,000 new cases of prostate cancer were discovered. According to the American Cancer Society, the estimated cases in 1996—just three years later—was 317,000, an increase of almost 100 percent.

Does this mean we are in the grips of a new prostate cancer epidemic?

No. Some of the increase is due to the fact that as the general population ages, the number of middle-aged and elderly men in the country is rising. Some is due to greater awareness of the disease among the population, coupled with better methods for earlier detection, including the increasing use of prostate-specific antigen (PSA) testing and digital rectal examination (DRE) to screen for asymptomatic prostate cancer; and some is due to improved diagnostic techniques, including the biopsy gun and ultrasound (see chapter 4).

Even though the incidence of prostate cancer is on the rise, so are survival rates. For this reason, the increased rate of diagnosis of prostate cancer should not be a cause for despair, but a signal for hope, because many of these tumors are now being detected in their earliest stages, when there is the best chance for cure.

Without early diagnosis and proper treatment, however, prostate cancer will remain a major killer. Over 41,000 American men will die of prostate cancer in 1996. The only cancer that causes more deaths among men is lung cancer, which killed 95,400 men in 1995. When all causes of death are considered, including everything from heart attack to murder, prostate cancer is responsible for three out of every 100 deaths of men in the United States.

MICROSCOPIC (AUTOPSY) CANCER VERSUS CLINICALLY APPARENT CANCER

Autopsy studies of the incidence of prostate cancer in men who have died of other causes have shown that many men have *microscopic disease*. This means that cancerous cells can be seen under a microscope, but the man never had any signs or symptoms that would have suggested a diagnosis of prostate cancer.

Clinically apparent disease is prostate cancer that is diagnosed during a man's lifetime. There is no way of knowing whether microscopic cancer would have progressed into clinically apparent prostate cancer, since no one knows what causes cancer to progress.

RISK FACTORS

Age

Age is the most important risk factor for prostate cancer, and every man over age forty is at risk. More than 80 percent of prostate cancers are diagnosed in men over age sixty-five, and more than 90 percent of the deaths from prostate cancer occur in this age group. In other words, the longer a man lives, the greater his risk of developing prostate cancer.

At least 20 percent of men in their sixties and more than 40 percent of men in their seventies harbor prostate cancer that is so small that it causes no symptoms. By age eighty, the number rises to 80 percent. For many years, these numbers were often cited as grounds for dismissing prostate cancer as just an "old man's disease," something inevitable and not worth treating aggressively. That is a dangerous myth. For one thing, it implies that precious research dollars and medical resources should not be wasted on older men.

The myth is also dangerous because it simply is untrue. As many as 30 percent of men in their thirties and forties—*three out*

Does Aging Cause Prostate Cancer?

Is there something about the process of aging itself that causes cancer? One intriguing possibility is that as we age, the immune system—the body's natural defense against infections and defective cells—begins to wear out.

Another possibility is that oxidative damage due to oxygen (*free radicals*) may trigger prostate cancer and other cancers. As we get older, our body may be less resistant to the damaging effects of these chemicals. Furthermore, the built-in repair mechanisms in the DNA of our cells may become less efficient at removing damaged bits of DNA and replacing them with normal DNA.

While these theories are being actively investigated, nothing has yet been proven.

---

of ten—have signs of precancer or already have cancer in their prostate. Fortunately, prostate cancer grows so slowly that there's a good chance these tumors, even in younger men, will not cause problems for many years—if ever.

Family History

Your genetic heritage also increases your chances of developing prostate cancer. If, say, your father had the disease, your own risk is about twice as high as a man with no family history of prostate cancer. The risk increases with the number of close family members who are affected: It is about five times greater if two relatives—your father and a brother, for example—have been affected, and up to eleven times greater if three relatives have it.

Another concern with familial prostate cancer is that it may be more likely to be fatal—not because the cancer is necessarily more aggressive, but because such tumors tend to become more active at a younger age, giving them more time to progress. For this reason, the American Cancer Society recommends that men with a family history of prostate cancer—on either their father's or their mother's side—should get an annual DRE and PSA beginning at age forty. Men without such a family history should get an annual DRE beginning at forty and an annual PSA after age fifty.

Scientists are trying to determine whether all men with prostate cancer have certain genes in common. Their goal is to identify *genetic markers*, specific patterns of DNA that might identify men at highest risk.

One marker that has attracted interest is the gene that's been named HPC1 (HPC stands for hereditary prostate cancer). Men who carry a certain form of the gene may have a high risk of getting prostate cancer. Even though the gene has been named, its exact location has not been found, and conflicting data refute the idea that HPC1 can predict cancer. At present there are no methods routinely available to screen for a high-risk form of HPC1, and only a small percentage of men carry it. There's no telling if and when HPC1 screening will ever prove useful for identifying high-risk men.

At the very least, research into HPC1 and other genetic markers may eventually help identify men who need earlier or more

---

PROSTATE CANCER AND YOUR MOTHER

No, your mother can't get prostate cancer . . . but you could have inherited from her certain genetic traits that increase your risk. When assessing risk, look at both branches of your family tree—all the male members on both your mother's and your father's side.

The presence of others in his family who have had prostate cancer does not mean a man (or his brothers, sons, grandsons, or nephews) is doomed. However, he should be especially vigilant. The American Cancer Society recommends that men with a family history of prostate cancer should start having a yearly PSA test and DRE at age forty.

frequent screening, more aggressive treatment, or closer monitoring, or those who would be candidates for chemoprevention trials (see page 45). Ideally, it will lead to a cure. Such results, however, are far down the scientific road.

Even if a genetic marker is found, it will not solve the entire problem of identifying who is at risk. Heredity is an important risk factor, but it is not the only one.

Ethnicity

Racial background seems to have a powerful effect on the risk of prostate cancer. African-American men, in particular, have the highest rate of prostate cancer of any group in the world: the incidence is 32 percent higher in American blacks than in American whites. Prostate cancer also develops earlier in African-American men. They are twice as likely as white men to get the disease when they are still in their early fifties.

Different ethnic groups have different rates of prostate cancer. Native Americans, Mexican Americans, and Chinese Americans have lower rates than Americans whose ancestors came from northern Europe. Globally, the rate of prostate cancer is highest in North America and northwestern Europe; Japan and other parts of Asia have the lowest rates.

Why these differences exist is unknown, but researchers have discovered a paradox wherein may lie a clue: We know that it is only the rate of *clinically apparent* prostate cancer that changes from one population group to another; the rate of *microscopic* prostate cancer (as determined by autopsy) is roughly the same all over the world. When men move and become assimilated into a new culture, they gradually assume the same risk as the men who have lived in that culture all their lives. For example, two generations after Japanese men move to the United States, their risk for having clinically apparent prostate cancer approaches that of white American males. Similarly, the death rate from prostate cancer for black males in the United States far exceeds that of black males in East Africa. Clearly, race is not the whole story. We need to look elsewhere for additional factors.

Environment

Something in the culture or environment of the industrialized Western world seems to convert microscopic prostate tumors into more aggressive, potentially fatal prostate cancer. Most likely, cancer results from a complex interaction of factors, including genetic susceptibility, diet, and exposure to *carcinogens*, substances that promote cancer. (Interestingly, the dog is the only animal that develops prostate cancer, and it is exposed to the same domestic environment as man.)

Some studies have suggested that certain occupations are associated with a slight increase in the risk of prostate cancer. Higher death rates have been reported in farmers, mechanics, and men who work with metals or rubber manufacturing. Workers exposed to cadmium, a trace mineral found in cigarette smoke and alkaline batteries, may be at increased risk, especially if they also smoke, but the findings are inconclusive.

Studies that look for trends cannot take into account all the possible variables that may contribute to cancer risk. For example, are farmers and manufacturing workers at higher risk because of their work, or because men in these professions tend to eat a higher-fat diet or smoke more than other men? Until these questions are answered, the jury is still out on the question of environmental risk. For now, our advice is not to worry about occupational exposure. If there is increased risk, it is quite small.

Sun Exposure

A man's risk may be influenced by where he lives. Prostate cancer rates are highest in the areas of the world that get the least amount of sun. In the United States, rates are highest in the northeastern states of New England and lowest in the Sunbelt states.

Why should this be so? Some evidence suggests that prostate cancer rates are higher in men who have low vitamin D levels. Sunlight is the major factor in vitamin D production, because ultraviolet (UV) radiation from the sun stimulates the body to manufacture vitamin D in the skin. It has been postulated that vitamin D, which appears to inhibit the growth of tumors, somehow prevents microscopic prostate cancer from progressing.

If you live in Maine, don't start packing your bags, and don't buy a lifetime membership in your neighborhood tanning parlor. The link between vitamin D and prostate cancer is still being studied. Besides, overexposure to UV radiation is a major cause of skin cancer. Your body needs only a little UV exposure to make all the vitamin D it needs.

You can also get vitamin D from your diet by eating foods such as fish and vitamin D–fortified milk. But avoid megadose supplements, since high doses of vitamin D can be toxic.

Hormones

The male hormone testosterone appears to be an essential factor in prostate cancer. The main source of testosterone is the testicles; studies find that men whose testicles were damaged or removed before puberty almost never develop prostate cancer. In addition, laboratory tests show that prostate cancer can be induced in rats by giving them testosterone for long periods of time.

Still, the precise nature of the relationship between testosterone and prostate cancer has not been defined. Virtually all men produce testosterone, but not all men develop prostate cancer.

Some evidence suggests that the role of hormones may explain some of the ethnic variations in the risk of prostate cancer. Different ethnic groups have different levels of testosterone. Studies show that African-American men generally have higher levels than do whites and they are at much higher risk for prostate cancer. Dutch men, whose risk is about the same as white American men, have higher testosterone levels than do Japanese men, a group that is at very low risk.

A hormone that travels through the bloodstream, called insulin-like growth factor-1, or IGF-1, has been linked to a higher risk for prostate cancer. IGF-1 is a powerful molecule that stimulates the growth of normal and cancerous prostate cells. Early testing shows that men with high levels of IGF-1 are more than four times as likely to get prostate cancer. Just as a high cholesterol level has become a red flag alerting people to watch for signs and symptoms of heart disease, a high IGF-1 level may one day become a warning sign for men who should be closely monitored for signs of prostate cancer. IGF-1 is a promising new marker, and scientists are actively investigating it. Before IGF-1 becomes a routine prostate cancer screening test, scientists must conduct a great deal more research to verify that it can live up to its billing as a reliable marker.

Diet

Diets that are high in fat, particularly fat from red meat, have also been implicated. A Harvard University study reported that men who eat a high-fat diet have a 79 percent increase in their risk. Conversely, a high-fiber, low-fat diet is associated with lower risk. Ethnic groups that eat relatively low-fat diets (Japanese, for example) also have a low incidence of prostate cancer.

Another dietary factor that has been proposed is beta carotene, a natural substance that is found in fruits and vegetables and that the body converts into vitamin A. In laboratory studies, vitamin A has been shown to inhibit the growth of cancer cells. Studies have also shown that people whose diets include lots of foods rich in beta carotene have relatively low levels of heart disease and cancer. As a result, many people assumed that taking beta carotene supplements could prevent disease.

Unfortunately, the beta carotene theory is not holding up under scrutiny. Multiple recent studies reported the disappointing finding—confirmed in subsequent research—that the substance was completely ineffective as a cancer preventive and may actually have increased risk slightly. Why? One explanation is that protection against cancer results from the complex interaction of hundreds of substances in a diet that is rich in fruits and vegetables, rather than from a single nutrient alone. Another possibility is that people who eat plenty of salads also eat less saturated fat. And they may be healthier to begin with. For example, perhaps the salad-bar set is likely to exercise more, smoke less, and drink more moderately than the meat-and-potatoes crowd. While there is no solid evidence that weighing too much, being out of shape, or drinking too much can cause prostate cancer, common sense tells us these factors probably don't help.

Vitamin E may also play a role in prostate cancer prevention. When a large group of men in Europe took 50 mg of vitamin E supplements every day for about six years, their chances of getting prostate cancer dropped significantly. If additional research confirms the anticancer effects of vitamin E, men will have an abundant, inexpensive preventive measure to help keep the disease at bay, However, the evidence is far from conclusive, and further investigation needs to be done. For one thing, the study wasn't even designed to measure the effects of vitamin E on prostate cancer: those findings were secondary. Also, all of the men in the study were white and smoked cigarettes, so the results may not have the same implications for nonsmokers or more diverse populations, such as African-Americans.

Fructose, the type of sugar found in fruit, may also have a protective effect. In one study, men who consumed five or more servings of fruit per day were half as likely to develop advanced prostate cancer as were men who ate less than one serving per day.

The same study indicated that too much calcium in the diet may increase the risk for prostate cancer. If that turns out to be true, someday men may be advised to limit their intake of dairy products and calcium supplements.

Several other studies suggest that the mineral selenium may reduce the risk of prostate cancer.

Should you run out and buy large bottles of vitamin E capsules, stop drinking milk, and order fruit salad every time you go out to eat? Let's put it this way: There's simply not enough evidence yet to conclude with certainty that vitamin E will make any difference when it comes to prostate cancer. But taking moderate amounts of it daily can do no harm and has been shown to have other beneficial effects, such as decreasing the risk of heart disease. The same goes for the findings about fructose and calcium, which are very new and unconfirmed, though you can't go wrong by increasing the amount of fresh fruit you consume, and vitamin C is essential in a balanced diet.

Unlikely Factors

Many other risk factors for prostate cancer have been proposed over the years, but scientists have not been able to find any proof that they make a difference. Here's a rundown:

VASECTOMY

Several years ago, the media devoted a lot of attention to a research report showing that the rate of prostate cancer seemed to be higher in men who had vasectomies—the contraceptive procedure in which the tubes that carry sperm from the testicles to the urethra are tied off. This was alarming news for the millions of men who had undergone the procedure.

What the media *didn't* spend a lot of time discussing was the fact that the statistical association between vasectomy and prostate cancer was weak, and that other studies did not show a link at all. Furthermore, there is no convincing biological explanation of why vasectomy would have any effect, either negative or positive, on prostate cancer. Still, people were concerned, so the National Institutes of Health (NIH) asked a panel of experts to review all the evidence.

WHO IS REALLY AT RISK?

What's the bottom line on risk factors? Are men in high-risk groups destined to develop prostate cancer? Are men from low-risk groups off the hook?

The answer to both questions is no.

All men are at risk for developing prostate cancer and should be screened regularly. Personal risk factors affect only how soon and how often one should have a checkup. Unfortunately, African-American men, who have an unusually high risk, have tended not to participate in voluntary screening programs. It is hoped that this situation will change in the near future as more people become aware of the importance of diagnosing prostate disease.

Their verdict?

Any increase in the rate of prostate cancer in men with vasectomy is probably due to "detection bias." In other words, men with vasectomies have seen doctors, so they are more likely than the overall population to have been screened for prostate cancer. And more screenings mean more detection of the disease.

Since vasectomy is unlikely to cause prostate cancer, the panel stated that there is no reason for men who have had vasectomies to have them reversed, nor is there any need for these men to be screened any sooner or more frequently than men who have not had vasectomies.

SMOKING

Smoking has not been strongly linked to prostate cancer. Many find that surprising because smoking has been implicated in so many other forms of cancer and, as noted above, because cigarette smoke contains cadmium. Of course, the lack of a strong connection does not mean that smoking is not harmful. Cigarettes and other forms of tobacco contain hundreds of toxic chemicals that can harm every cell in the body—not just the lungs, throat, and mouth.

BENIGN PROSTATIC HYPERPLASIA (BPH)

Logically, BPH might seem to be linked to prostate cancer. The two conditions do have a number of similarities: Both depend on hormonal stimulation from testosterone, and both are more likely to develop as a man ages. They can even cause similar symptoms. Furthermore, the two conditions may exist at the same time. So far, however, no direct link between the two has been found. It may simply be that, as in the case of vasectomy, there is an increased likelihood that men who see doctors for BPH treatment will have their cancer detected.

SEXUAL BEHAVIOR

Perhaps it is natural for men to wonder if the number of orgasms they have in their lifetime is related to their risk of prostate cancer. Since the prostate produces part of the seminal fluid, some people theorize that not having frequent regular orgasms to expel the fluid can cause it to "back up" inside the gland, leading to prostate cancer.

This is false. For one thing, semen does not accumulate. The body produces the amount it needs and holds on to it for a while. If it is not ejaculated within a certain period of time, it is reabsorbed by the body and a fresh supply is produced.

It would be more logical to infer that having too much sex would increase risk. Men who become sexually active when they are very young and who have multiple sex partners are at increased risk for sexually transmitted diseases, and there is some evidence that sexually transmitted diseases are associated with genital cancers in women—but so far, no such link has been found for prostate cancer.

VIRUSES

Viruses are associated with the development of some kinds of cancer. It is likely, however, that viruses are just one of many triggers, and there is no evidence of specific viruses that are involved in prostate cancer. Bear in mind, though, that cancers do not "spread" from one person to another like a contagious disease.

SOCIOECONOMIC FACTORS

Factors such as income and educational level have also been explored as possible risk factors. But if a link is ever found, it is likely to be indirect. In other words, one assumes that people with more money are more likely to take better care of themselves and eat a healthy diet, which in turn could have an impact on the rate of prostate cancer.

PREVENTION

There is nothing a man can do about the major known risk factors for prostate cancer: age, genetics, and ethnicity. As long as he's alive, he'll continue to get older. He can't change the genes he inherited from his parents, and he can't change his ethnic identity.

Certain dietary factors may increase the risk for prostate cancer, but the evidence in favor of or against any specific dietary component is not strong enough to result in firm recommendations. At this point, the most prudent course of action is to eat a well-balanced diet, choose most of the foods you eat from plant sources, and limit your intake of high-fat foods, particularly those that come from animals.

Researchers are investigating a number of chemical substances, including drugs and vitamins, that may someday prove useful in preventing cancer. This approach, called *chemoprevention*, is also aimed at trying to halt or slow the progression of cancer in high-risk individuals. One major study, the Prostate Cancer Prevention Trial (PCPT), is being conducted to determine whether the drug finasteride (Proscar), currently used to treat BPH, might be of value as chemoprevention for prostate cancer. Finasteride lowers the level of the hormone dihydrotestosterone, or DHT, which causes benign prostate enlargement. Although finasteride may not actually prevent prostate cancer, the study hopes to determine whether it can have a role in inhibiting the progression of clinically significant disease.

The PCPT study, one of the largest chemoprevention studies ever conducted, was organized by the U.S. government's principal agency for cancer research, the National Cancer Institute, in 1993. The trial, expected to last for ten years, will involve at least eighteen thousand men aged fifty-five years and older. For more information about the study, call the NCI's Cancer Information Service at 1-800-4-CANCER (1-800-422-6237).

Chapter 4

How Is Prostate Cancer Detected?

Prostate cancer begins slowly and silently. A single cancerous cell *doubles*—that is, it reproduces itself by division. One cell becomes two; two become four, and so on. After doubling about thirty to thirty-five times, the cells form a tumor one cubic centimeter in size (about as big as half a peanut). It is not until this point that a physical exam may detect the tumor.

Early detection is crucial, because the window of opportunity for detecting curable prostate cancer is small. The tumor spends about 70 percent of its life span growing to a size that is considered clinically significant. Once it grows beyond that point, it becomes progressively more likely to produce symptoms, spread to adjacent and distant sites, and perhaps even cause death.

The good news—and the best reason to have regular checkups—is that prostate cancer, if found soon enough, can usually be cured.

In this chapter, we describe the tests for diagnosing and evaluating prostate cancer. Not all of these tests are necessary for every man with prostate cancer. Your doctor will recommend the ones that are appropriate for you.

SYMPTOMS AND SIGNS

Symptoms are disease-related problems that you experience; *signs* are outward manifestations that someone else can observe or measure. Pain is a symptom; feeling a lump in the prostate is a sign. Unfortunately, early prostate cancer does not usually cause symptoms (see chapter 2, p. 29). Unless the tumor begins very close to the urethra and interferes with the flow of urine, it probably will not cause symptoms until it has grown quite large or spread beyond the prostate.

When urinary symptoms occur, they are usually similar to those seen in conditions such as benign prostatic hyperplasia (BPH). The only difference may be that symptoms often develop more slowly when they are caused by BPH.

Symptoms may include changes in voiding pattern—for example, slowing or weakening of the urinary stream, having the need to urinate more frequently or more urgently, or feeling that the bladder is not emptying well. The only way to determine what is causing the problem is by physical examination of the prostate and by diagnostic tests. A man should consult a doctor if he no-

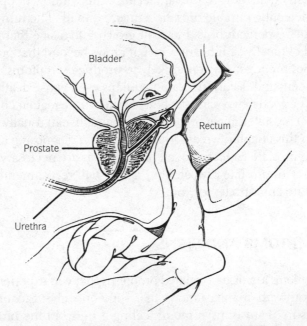

Figure 4.1: Digital rectal examination (DRE).

tices blood in his urine or semen, or there is a decrease in the amount of fluid he ejaculates. These are not common symptoms of cancer, but they may indicate that the urethra or ejaculatory ducts are blocked. Impotence or less rigid erections also may develop in late cancer if the tumor invades the nerves involved in erection, but this is uncommon. If the cancer has metastasized, the lymph nodes may be swollen or there may be pain in such areas as the spine, ribs, hips, or pelvis.

Many prostate cancer symptoms are *nonspecific*—in other words, the same problems can arise in a number of other medical conditions. There is no way of pinpointing the exact cause of a certain symptom without a thorough diagnostic evaluation. In any case, men should not wait to see a doctor until symptoms develop—by then it may be too late to attempt a cure. The best approach is to have regular checkups that include a prostate exam so the cancer can be found as early as possible.

DIGITAL RECTAL EXAMINATION (DRE)

This simple, brief physical examination of the prostate is the cornerstone of prostate cancer detection. It may be uncomfortable, even embarrassing for some, and it is not foolproof. But it is essential for monitoring the health of the prostate. The American Cancer Society recommends that every man over the age of forty have a DRE every year as part of a routine annual checkup.

The prostate's location, next to the rectum near the anal opening, makes it possible for doctors to feel it by inserting a lubricated, gloved finger into the rectum and pressing toward the pubic bone (Fig. 4.1). During the DRE, depending on the doctor's preference, the patient may be asked to stand and bend forward over the examining table, or he may kneel or lie on the table on his side. The entire procedure takes only about a minute.

Normally, the surface of the prostate is smooth and elastic—it has been described as feeling like the tip of your nose. As the doc-

tor palpates the prostate, he or she is feeling for lumps, enlargement, or anything else abnormal. A cancerous lesion often starts
as a small, hard bump or nodule; as the cancer develops, this nodule grows larger, and more lumps may appear.

While in some cases a doctor may be able to detect whether
the cancer has spread outside the prostate, invading the seminal
vesicles or the side wall of the pelvis, the DRE has limitations.
First, the doctor can feel only the back (posterior) wall of the
gland. Fortunately, that is where most prostate cancers begin.
Second, it is difficult to feel cancer nodules that are very small or
that are deep inside the prostate. Third, any prostate enlargement
due to BPH can "cushion" or obscure the cancer nodules so they
cannot be felt. The net result is that DRE will miss as many as 50
percent of prostate cancers. This is one reason many men already
have advanced disease before DRE detects cancer.

What can a man expect if his doctor does detect a hard or suspicious area? He should not panic. Fewer than half of the nodules
detected by DRE turn out to be cancerous. Such results, called
false positives, may arise because other abnormalities are present,
including BPH, stones, prostate infections, and lesions from pre-
vious surgery of the prostate. Once a suspicious area is found,
however, further testing is always needed to establish a diagnosis.

Despite its limitations, DRE should not be neglected or
avoided. It remains the first line of defense against prostate cancer.

PROSTATE-SPECIFIC ANTIGEN (PSA) TEST

Prostate-specific antigen is a protein molecule that is produced
almost exclusively by cells in the prostate. This enzyme is normally present in low amounts in the blood. (To be precise, PSA is
found in the *serum*, which is the clear fluid component of blood.)
When a problem arises in the prostate, more PSA leaks into the
bloodstream. Factors that can increase PSA concentration include cancer, infections, and BPH.

The blood test for measuring PSA is one of the most valuable tools available for the diagnosis of prostate cancer.* PSA tests can detect nearly twice as many prostate cancers as DRE alone. Even more important, about two thirds of the cancers detected by the test are still confined to the prostate—meaning that they have the best chance of a cure.

Any primary-care physician can order a PSA test, which is often done along with other routine blood work. The results are usually available within one to three days. It should be stressed that PSA results do not confirm whether or not prostate cancer is present. The test is simply a signpost, pointing either toward or away from the diagnosis.

The normal range for serum PSA is 0.0 to 4.0 ng/mL (nanograms per milliliter), but the range varies with age. As a man gets older, what we consider a normal PSA increases slightly. For this reason, many doctors now advocate using "age adjusted" cutoffs for the ranges of PSA considered normal and abnormal. In other words, a PSA level of 3.0 ng/mL might be normal for a 50-year-old man, while 6.5 ng/mL might be normal at age 80. The discrepancy reflects the fact that so many men tend to develop BPH as they age, and BPH is one of the many conditions that can elevate PSA.

While PSA results are not exact, they can reflect the stage of cancer. The higher the PSA value, the greater the chance that a tumor has progressed and spread beyond the prostate. Test results can also help a man and his doctor decide on the best course of treatment. A very high PSA level can indicate that the cancer has spread out into the lymph nodes.

PSA tests also indicate the response to treatment. If the cancer is eradicated by surgery or radiation, or controlled by hormone therapy, the PSA level will fall to practically zero; ideally, it will

---

* PSA has just about replaced the older test, for prostatic acid phosphatase (PAP). Another blood test detects a substance called *alkaline phosphatase*, which increases when the bones are growing rapidly, as in cases of metastatic cancer. But the test is not very accurate or specific for prostate cancer, so it too is hardly used any more.

WHAT AFFECTS SERUM PSA LEVELS?

Some of the causes of an elevated PSA are:

- Prostate cancer
- Recent prostate biopsy
- Recent prostate surgery
- Benign prostatic hyperplasia (BPH)
- Urinary tract infection
- Prostatitis (prostate infection)
- Stones in the prostate
- Vigorous prostate massage (but not DRE)
- Aging (may be related to BPH)

If a condition is reversed (for example, if a urinary tract infection is cleared up), the PSA level should return to normal.

Certain medications, notably finasteride (Proscar) and other agents that lower testosterone levels, can cause the PSA level to fall.

be completely undetectable—less than 0.1 ng/mL. If it increases significantly again later, it is possible that the cancer has recurred.

In dealing with PSA results, remember that the PSA test is not 100 percent accurate. A low PSA level does not necessarily mean you are cancer-free, and a high PSA level does not absolutely mean you have cancer. Many factors can influence PSA levels, and your situation is not the same as anyone else's. Keeping a PSA diary may help you put your PSA results in perspective.

Prostate cancer does *not always* cause the PSA level to rise. Up to a third of prostate cancers that are still confined to the prostate produce a normal serum PSA level. In these cases, the level might go up over time but still stay within the borderline range.

Interpreting the results of a PSA test is sometimes difficult, especially when levels are in the borderline range between 4.0 and 10.0 ng/mL. Like the DRE, the PSA test sometimes produces false positive results. This means many men who do not have can-

---

PUTTING PSA IN PERSPECTIVE

PSA alone cannot reveal all cases of prostate cancer.

About one fifth of men with prostate cancer have "normal" PSA levels (less than 4.0 ng/mL); about the same number have PSA levels in the "borderline" range (4.0 to 10.0 ng/mL). In addition, about one third of men with high PSA levels (over 10 ng/mL) turn out not to have cancer.

Nor can DRE alone reveal all prostate cancers. But when the two tests are done together, they detect the majority of prostate cancers. If one is abnormal and the other is not, additional tests are necessary.

---

cer may experience a brief period of additional testing and worry. For the more fortunate, a little anxiety may be forgotten with the assurance that they are cancer-free. For the men who do have prostate cancer, however, the PSA test may be life-saving.

Recent refinements in PSA testing have helped make results more accurate. One of these, PSA *density*, or PSAD, measures the correlation between the PSA level and the size and weight of the prostate as estimated by ultrasound examination. PSAD can help the doctor determine, for example, whether a PSA elevation results from cancer or from BPH. In BPH, the increase in the PSA level generally corresponds to the amount of prostatic enlargement. In cancer, the PSA level may increase out of proportion to the size of the prostate.

PSAD, while promising, is currently limited by the accuracy of the ultrasound, which often depends on who conducts the examination. Some researchers have found no advantages to the PSAD over regular PSA testing.

PSA *velocity* is a measurement of the trend of change in PSA levels over time. This test reflects the fact that the actual PSA number may not be as important as the *changes* in that level from one test to the next. By analyzing how rapidly the serum PSA level rises or falls, it may be possible to predict whether a man is likely to have prostate cancer.

While PSA velocity may prove useful for discovering cancer in some men, it has some practical drawbacks. For one, PSA test results can vary if different laboratories are used to conduct the blood analyses. In addition, determining a change in velocity requires results from three PSA tests taken over at least two years. This means the doctor must delay treatment decisions based on velocity for a relatively long time.

The most exciting news in prostate cancer diagnosis may be the free PSA test. Normally, some of the PSA enzyme is chemically attached (bound or *complexed*) to other proteins circulating in the blood. The rest stays free, circulating in its unbound form. While the regular PSA test determines the level of total PSA (free PSA and complexed PSA combined), the free PSA test detects only the level of the free form. Knowing the level of free PSA is important, because men with prostate cancer have a lower value than those without cancer. The lower the ratio of free PSA to total PSA, the higher the likelihood that a patient has cancer and not BPH.

Some doctors claim that the new test will eliminate the need for biopsies for some men, but others strongly disagree. Even though the free PSA test promises a much greater degree of accuracy than the regular PSA test, it can still give "false negative" results, meaning it may indicate that no cancer is present when in fact a tumor exists. For now, the greatest value of the free PSA test is as a follow-up for men with borderline total PSA scores, say from 2.5 to 10.0 ng/mL. Results from the free PSA test will help doctors decide when a biopsy is necessary.

Variations on the PSA Test

Reverse transcriptase-polymerase chain reaction, or RT-PCR, is a method for detecting small amounts of RNA, a substance related to DNA that is needed for cells to produce proteins. There are specific RNAs for each protein in the body. The RT-PCR test for prostate cancer cells looks specifically for the RNA sequence that is responsible for making PSA. A potential advantage of this test is that it can detect very small numbers of prostate cancer cells in the blood that would be missed by other tests. The disadvantage is that doctors are still not sure whether having a few prostate cancer cells in the bloodstream means a man will actually develop distant metastases that grow enough to cause other symptoms or affect survival.

Most studies of RT-PCR have looked into its use for men who already have prostate cancer. The test may be useful before treatment to help determine which options are most suitable or to help in the early detection of recurrent cancer. For now, RT-PCR is not recommended as a screening test for early cancer diagnosis.

The proteins hK2 and prostate-specific membrane antigen (PMSA) are related to PSA, and both are under scrutiny as possible markers for prostate cancer. The roles of these molecules in cancer diagnosis or for monitoring patients during treatment is uncertain, and none are in routine use, though several groups are vigorously investigating them.

TRANSRECTAL ULTRASOUND (TRUS)

If a DRE or PSA test indicates a problem may exist, the doctor will probably suggest ultrasound as the next step. Transrectal (the word means "through the rectum") ultrasound, also called sonography, is a valuable imaging technique. Using harmless sound waves and their echoes to "map" the prostate, TRUS produces a detailed picture of the entire prostate, revealing its size and the presence of abnormalities.

TRUS is usually done by a specialist (either a urologist or a radiologist) in the office or in an outpatient clinic. With the patient lying on his side, a slim, wand-shaped probe is inserted into the rectum. This probe emits high-frequency sound waves that bounce off the prostate and back to the probe. A computer translates the echoes into images on a video screen (Fig. 4.2).

A typical TRUS examination takes about twenty minutes. The procedure is painless, but since insertion of the probe can be un-

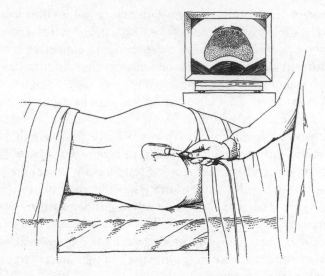

Figure 4.2: Transrectal ultrasound (TRUS) procedure.

comfortable for a few seconds, an anesthetic lubricating jelly may be used to ease the discomfort.

TRUS may be done for different reasons at different points in the diagnosis and treatment of prostate cancer. The first time is usually because something abnormal was found during DRE or PSA testing, or because a man with a high prostate cancer risk has developed symptoms. There is no reason to have TRUS when both the DRE and PSA are normal.

TRUS can sometimes identify cancer that cannot be felt by DRE, and it may give a good picture of cancerous nodules. For that reason, the procedure is often used during a biopsy to help the physician locate and sample tissue. Many newer TRUS units have a biopsy needle guide built right in, so the biopsy can be done directly through the probe. This is a major advance over "blind" biopsies, in which the doctor uses a fingertip to guide the needle.

As do all diagnostic tests, TRUS has its limitations. In some men, the ultrasound cannot detect a difference between abnormal cancerous tissue and normal prostate tissue, nor can it always distinguish between cancerous and noncancerous lumps. Diffuse cancers are more difficult to visualize than solid, nodular tumors, and may not be revealed by ultrasound. Even so, TRUS is a valuable diagnostic tool.

BIOPSY

A biopsy is an essential step in the diagnosis of prostate cancer. Small samples of tissue are removed from the prostate and examined under a microscope. The biopsy is used to determine the *Gleason score*, a critical element in predicting the aggressiveness of an individual cancer (see chapter 5 for more information).

Less than ten years ago, prostate biopsies often had to be done in the hospital under general anesthesia. Today, most biopsies are done as an outpatient procedure, usually in the urologist's office. With modern equipment, there usually is no need for anesthesia or sedation, and the entire procedure takes only a few minutes.

The doctor typically takes a sample using a specially designed biopsy needle that captures a tiny sliver, or *core*, of tissue. This needle is inserted into the prostate through the rectum (*transrectal biopsy*). The *biopsy gun*—a spring-loaded, trigger-activated device—precisely targets small areas of abnormal tissue. Because it uses a relatively small needle and takes samples in less than a second, it causes little discomfort. Biopsies are often done using transrectal ultrasound (Fig. 4.3), which lets the doctor clearly see the areas that need to be sampled. It is also possible to do finger-guided biopsies. Some doctors will also biopsy the seminal vesicles at the same time.

Biopsy cores are taken from several different areas of the prostate to get a representative sampling of the entire gland. A *sex-*

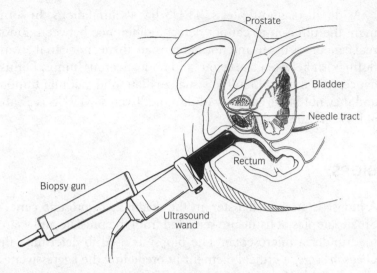

Figure 4.3: Prostate biopsy using the biopsy gun.

tant biopsy takes six samples, from the apex (the end farthest from the bladder), the middle, and the base (the end closest to the bladder) of both the right and left sides of the prostate gland. The doctor will also take samples directly from any suspicious lesions.

After the procedure, the tissue samples are sent to a lab. There, a pathologist examines the biopsy cores under a microscope to look for abnormal cells and determine whether they are cancerous. In his report, the pathologist will note what proportion of a biopsy contains cancer, what grade the cancer is, and whether the cancerous cells are invading surrounding tissue. This report, combined with the results of other diagnostic tests—including PSA level, DRE, and TRUS—and symptoms, provides as clear a picture as possible of the patient's clinical situation and helps his doctor determine treatment options.

As with all other diagnostic methods, biopsies have some shortcomings. Sometimes cancer is present, but the biopsy needle misses it completely. This is known as a *sampling error*, and about 15 percent of the time it is responsible for a false-negative result—in other words, the man has cancer that did not show up on the biopsy. Also, the biopsy may not reveal the full extent of the cancer: The sampled tissue may show there is only a small amount of cancer when there is actually a lot in other, unsampled parts of the prostate.

The biopsy can be uncomfortable and it is not a procedure many men would want to undergo frequently. You may feel a stinging sensation each time the biopsy needle pierces the prostate, but any soreness or discomfort passes quickly. Biopsy does *not* increase the chance that the cancer will spread, but like all surgical procedures, it does pose some risks. Serious bleeding and infection are very rare, but minor bleeding is relatively common. For a week or so afterward, you may see small amounts of blood in your urine, semen, or bowel movements. Alert your doctor immediately if the bleeding is heavy or prolonged.

To prevent bleeding, your doctor may ask you to stop taking any medications that interfere with blood clotting, such as aspirin or Coumadin, before the biopsy.

To prevent infection, which can develop if the biopsy needle transmits germs from the rectum into the prostate, most men have an enema before the biopsy and take antibiotics before and after the procedure. Signs of infection include pain on urination, discharge from the penis, or fever. *Sepsis*—infection in the bloodstream, causing high fever—is rare but serious. Alert your doctor immediately if any of these problems arise.

Another rare complication is swelling of the prostate and difficulty urinating, which can lead to urinary retention. If your bladder is unable to empty, it may be necessary for your doctor to place a tube, or catheter, in the urethra to let the urine drain out.

OTHER DIAGNOSTIC TECHNIQUES

During a workup for prostate cancer, your doctor may ask you to undergo certain nonsurgical tests that produce images of the inside of your body. The following section describes these tests in order of how frequently they are used.

Bone Scan

The main purpose of a bone scan is to see if prostate cancer has spread to the bones. Radioactive material is injected into a vein, where it circulates in the bloodstream and is absorbed by the bones. The injected material makes the bones show up more clearly and more accurately on the film. Cancer that has metastasized to bones causes rapid bone growth. The radioactive agent concentrates in those growth sites, showing up on film as "hot spots." Bone scans often detect cancer spread earlier than regular X rays. Keep in mind that if you've ever had back surgery, arthritis, or broken bones, these sites can also appear as hot spots. If the bone scan reveals hot spots, further tests, such as regular X rays or *magnetic resonance imaging* (described below) may be done to get a more detailed picture of the bone.

Bone scans are neither painful nor uncomfortable and are usually done on an outpatient basis in a hospital or radiology clinic. The amount of radioactivity involved is very small and safe. Bone scans do not increase the risk of other cancers, nor do they harm the bones or any other organs. Any leftover material is excreted in the urine.

CT Scan

CT, or *computerized tomography*, is a series of X rays taken by a machine that rotates all the way around your body. A computer translates the information into a detailed cross-sectional view of your insides. For better results, you may be given a *contrast medium*, a dye that is injected or swallowed to make the organs show up in sharp contrast.

CT scanning is painless, and the radiation exposure is minimal, but the procedure, which takes up to an hour, can be tedious. You lie on a flat table that slowly moves you through the scanner, which looks like a giant ring. In some cases the contrast medium can cause adverse reactions: diarrhea from the liquid dye, and sensations of warmth or flushing, itching, and even hives from the intravenous dye. Serious allergic reactions are rare, but you should tell the radiotherapist before the procedure if you have allergies.

Most men get a CT scan before beginning radiation therapy to help the radiotherapist plan how much radiation to deliver and where to direct it. Occasionally a CT scan is done to see whether cancer has spread to the lymph nodes, but the technique is not reliable for this purpose (a lymph node dissection is the better approach; see chapter 8 for more information).

MRI

Magnetic resonance imaging (MRI) is a noninvasive diagnostic technique that uses powerful magnetic fields and radio frequency signals to create high-quality pictures. A scanner measures the specific amounts of magnetic energy given off by the various cells. Using this information, a computer constructs cross-sectional images of internal organs and tissues. MRI provides excellent images of the spinal cord, the brain, and the bones. In many cases an MRI is ordered to clarify the findings on a bone scan.

Like CT scanning, MRI is a slow process. You may have to stay in the scanner—a long, narrow, and noisy tunnel—for an hour. There is no pain or discomfort with the procedure. You may be given a contrast agent to enhance the MRI images; adverse reactions to these substances are uncommon. Some patients find the noise inside the tunnel disconcerting. Most doctors will prescribe a short-acting oral sedative to alleviate any anxiety. Recently a new form of MRI, called *open-air MRI*, has become available in some centers. As the name suggests, this machine eliminates the tunnel and reduces the "closed-in" feeling.

Intravenous pyelogram (IVP)

For an *intravenous pyelogram*, or *IVP* (also called a *urogram*), an iodine dye is injected into a vein in the arm. The dye gets filtered by the kidneys before being eliminated by the body; usually the dye does not cause any side effects. Before it is completely gone, X rays pick up the dye, which appears white on the film. An IVP yields a good picture of the structure and function of the kidneys, bladder, and ureter. Though it does not give any direct information about the prostate, it can show whether prostate cancer has had any effect on the urinary system. An IVP is more likely to be done as part of an initial routine evaluation of urinary symptoms than as part of a prostate cancer workup, since a CT or MRI scan will probably provide more useful information.

Cystoscopy

Cystoscopy is an examination of the inside of the urethra, prostate, and bladder using a long, thin instrument inserted through the urethra. Most men are surprised to find that cystoscopy is not painful—just a bit uncomfortable. Cystoscopy is often done to look for bladder cancer when blood is seen in the urine and can also help diagnose stones and other bladder abnormalities, but it is not usually part of the standard evaluation for prostate cancer.

SUMMARY

There is no single perfect method for detecting prostate cancer. However, a combination of DRE, PSA testing, and TRUS-guided biopsy offers the best chance of finding cancer while there is still time for a cure. If initial findings are ambiguous, more tests, such as repeat biopsies or further imaging studies, may be needed. Viewed in their entirety, the results of your clinical workup will help you and your caregiver make the best decisions about your future course of treatment.

Chapter 5

Grade and Stage:
What Do the Numbers Mean?

When the time comes to decide which treatment is best for you, knowing the grade and stage of your prostate cancer is essential. In simple terms, the *grade* indicates how aggressive the cancer is, and *stage* indicates the extent of its spread within the body. Together, these pieces of the puzzle show how aggressive the cancer is and how likely it is to have spread beyond the prostate.

In this chapter, we explain the *Gleason score*, which evaluates grade, and the *TNM system* of staging. Other systems, such as the Whitmore-Jewett staging system ("ABCD"), have also been used to describe prostate cancers, but the Gleason and the TNM—the most current and useful methods available—are rapidly becoming the standard scales of measurement worldwide.

BEWARE THE NUMBERS GAME

Before going further, some cautions:

Because prostate cancer develops inside the gland, hidden from direct view, no presurgical staging classification system can be 100 percent accurate. Your doctors will collect all the information they can before assigning a stage; this process is known as *clinical staging*. An assessment of the cancer based on microscopic analysis of tissue taken directly from the prostate or lymph nodes after surgery is called *pathologic staging*. The type and scope of the information gathered for clinical staging differs greatly from that gleaned through pathologic staging. It is not surprising to find that the two assessments may not agree. One possible result of this discrepancy is *understaging*, which occurs when tissues removed during surgery reveal more extensive cancer than earlier tests indicated. As Ralph, a sixty-one-year-old industrial chemist from Arizona put it, "I went from a B to a D on the operating table." This is a dramatic change which can be upsetting. But the microscopic examination of cancer cells and the pathologist's resulting report is the final word, the gold standard of staging. However, pathologic staging is possible only if the cancer is treated surgically, which is not always necessary or desirable.

Another (albeit minor) problem is that classification systems are constantly being refined. As we learn more about cancer and apply that knowledge to the diagnosis and the outcome of treatment, we keep fine-tuning the system so that it is increasingly accurate. Each change clarifies the clinical picture.

As you continue to read books and articles about prostate cancer, you will find many authors used the ABCD system, while more recent works adopt the TNM system. The conversion chart on page 68 should help you compare the two major staging systems.

GRADING

While there are other methods for grading prostate cancer, most doctors use the Gleason system, named after the doctor who developed it. The Gleason grade is based on the microscopic appearance of cells extracted by biopsy from the prostate. The pathologist decides on the grade of the tumor by studying the architecture of the cells—that is, their shape and arrangement.

The extent to which cancer cells (and the glandular structures they form) resemble in shape normal cells and glands is called *differentiation*. Well-differentiated cells vary only slightly from normal cells and form clearly identifiable glandular units. Poorly differentiated cells tend to merge together into a shapeless mass.

THE FIVE GLEASON GRADES

Grade 1: Cancer is well differentiated, composed of uniformly spaced circular acini in a circumscribed compact mass.

Grade 2: Cancer is still well differentiated, but acini are arranged more loosely and are more irregular in shape; some acini invade neighboring prostatic tissue.

Grade 3: Most common grade of prostate cancer; cancer is moderately differentiated, with acini varying in size from small to large; many acini invade neighboring prostatic tissue.

Grade 4: Cancer is poorly differentiated, unable to form separate acinar units; highly irregular, distorted shapes; progressive invasion of neighboring tissue.

Grade 5: Cancer is undifferentiated and bears no resemblance to normal prostate cells. Cells are unable to form acinar units.

The more poorly differentiated the cells are, the more aggressive and malignant they are (Fig. 5.1).

In assigning a Gleason score, the pathologist studies the sample and identifies the two most common cell patterns present. These are called the *primary* and *secondary* patterns. Then the pathologist assigns a Gleason grade between 1 (well differentiated) and 5 (poorly differentiated) to each of these patterns. The two grades are added together to produce the Gleason score, sometimes called the *Gleason sum.*

Here are some examples: If a pathologist assigns the primary pattern a grade of 2 and the secondary pattern a grade of 3, the combined Gleason score would be 5 (2+3). The lowest possible Gleason score is 2 (1+1) and the highest is 10 (5+5). Scores of 4 or less indicate low-grade prostate cancer. These well-differentiated cancers tend to be the slowest growing and the least dangerous. Intermediate-grade cancer, with Gleason scores of 5 and 6, is moderately differentiated. Gleason scores of 7 to 10 indicate high-grade cancer, which has poorly differentiated cells.

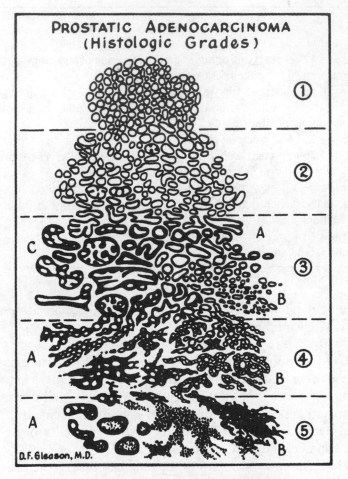

Figure 5.1: Appearance of cancer cells, ranked according to the Gleason grade.

High-grade cancer is often very aggressive and fast-growing, and it can be deadly.

As a rule, the lower your Gleason score, the better you are likely to do. The operative word here is *likely*: Remember, the Gleason score is a guideline, not a guarantee. The Gleason grade assesses only the results of the prostate biopsy, and, as discussed in chapter 4, biopsy studies themselves are not perfect. The needle may not have collected representative samples of cancer tissue. Accuracy is a particular problem with small, low-grade tumors, in which the needle is more likely to miss its target. *Sextant biopsies,* in which tissue is taken from six areas, three from each side of the prostate, can improve the chances for accuracy.

Keep in mind that your Gleason score is not the ultimate determinant of outcome; it needs to be seen in the context of other factors, including the tumor's stage.

STAGING SYSTEMS

The stage of a prostate cancer reflects the extent of the cancer: how big it is and whether it is contained inside the prostate. If it is not contained, the stage indicates where and how far it has spread. In prostate cancer, most staging numbers reflect *clinical* staging. *Pathologic* staging is only possible after radical prostatectomy, the surgical removal of the prostate.

Clinical staging of prostate cancer is more complex than grading because it combines several different parameters: results of digital rectal examination (DRE), PSA level, estimated tumor volume, Gleason score, and other tests that indicate whether the cancer has spread to the seminal vesicles, lymph nodes, or more distant tissues such as bones or the lungs.

The first factor is whether or not the tumor can be felt on DRE. Cancers that cannot be felt are called *nonpalpable.* Nonpalpable cancers may be discovered when part of the prostate is *resected* (surgically removed) during treatment for some problem other than cancer, such as benign prostatic hyperplasia (BPH). Nonpalpable cancers also may be detected by an elevated PSA level.

If a biopsy confirms prostate cancer, additional tests may be done. As discussed in chapter 4, these include bone scan, CT scan, magnetic resonance imaging, and other diagnostic

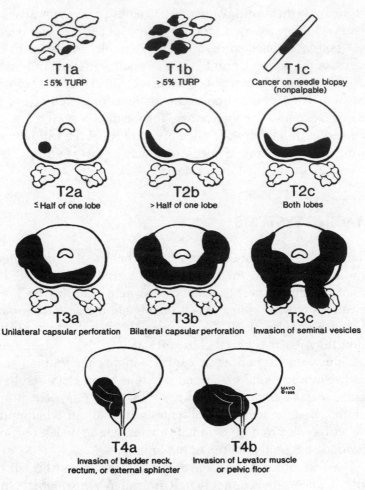

T1a
≤ 5% TURP

T1b
> 5% TURP

T1c
Cancer on needle biopsy
(nonpalpable)

T2a
≤ Half of one lobe

T2b
> Half of one lobe

T2c
Both lobes

T3a
Unilateral capsular perforation

T3b
Bilateral capsular perforation

T3c
Invasion of seminal vesicles

T4a
Invasion of bladder neck,
rectum, or external sphincter

T4b
Invasion of Levator muscle
or pelvic floor

*Figure 5.2: Extent of prostate cancer,
according to the TNM staging system.*

procedures that indicate whether the cancer has spread beyond the prostate.

The doctor, usually a urologist or an oncologist, reviews all the
results and determines the cancer stage.

TNM System

The TNM system is the international standard for staging cancer. The **T** refers to the extent of the original (primary) tumor in the prostate. The **N** refers to the status of the lymph nodes in the pelvic region; since these nodes are so close to the prostate, the cancer often spreads there first. The **M** refers to the presence or absence of distant metastasis—that is, whether the cancer has traveled out of the immediate area of the prostate to other parts of the body. Fig. 5.2 illustrates the extent of cancer as described by the TNM system.

Each T stage has substages numbered from 0 to 4 in increasing order of the relative seriousness of the clinical finding. The number 0 following a letter indicates that there is no evidence of that particular parameter. To be specific: T0 = no evidence of tumor; N0 = no regional lymph node metastasis; and M0 = no distant metastasis.

The tumor stages are further divided into substages by the letters a–c:

- Stages T1a–c: nonpalpable tumor
- Stages T2a–c: palpable tumor; confined to the prostate
- Stages T3a–c: tumor extending outside the prostate (T3a or b) or invading seminal vesicles (T3c)
- Stages T4a and b: tumor invading additional organs/tissues next to the prostate such as the bladder or rectum

Although the TNM system roughly corresponds to the older ABCD system, its subcategories are more detailed in describing the size and invasiveness of the tumor.

ABCD Staging System

In this system, prostate cancer is divided into four categories, each of which is divided into substages, depending on the extent and grade of the cancer (usually the Gleason score). Details of the substages appear in Table 5.1. The general categories are:

- Stage A: nonpalpable cancer found incidentally during TURP or adenomectomy
- Stage B: cancer found because of an abnormal DRE; confined to the prostate
- Stage C: cancer spread to tissues outside the prostate
- Stage D: metastasis to lymph nodes, bone, or other tissue

As Table 5.1 indicates, Stage A is roughly equivalent to T1, Stage B to T2, and Stage C to T3.

The advantage of the ABCD system is its relative simplicity. The disadvantage is that it is not very precise.

TOWARD MORE ACCURATE STAGING

Is clinical staging foolproof?

No. As with Gleason grading, the test results on which staging is based may not be completely accurate. As a consequence, prostate cancer is often *understaged*. Pathologic staging reveals that more than half of prostate cancers turn out to be more advanced than the clinical stage indicated. Only 5 percent turn out to have been *overstaged*—that is, there is less cancer than was indicated by the clinical stage. Despite these imperfections, we have no choice but to rely on clinical staging as a guide to initial therapy.

A number of recent approaches that may improve the accuracy of clinical staging are being studied. Some of the most promising new techniques include use of serum PSA with TRUS; sextant biopsies; estimation of tumor volume; flow cytometry and DNA ploidy; polymerase chain reaction for PSA-producing cells in blood; microvessel density; serum prostate-specific membrane antigen (PSM); and the Multiple Prognostic Index, which is a consistent, structured analysis of a combination of factors that helps predict outcome.

Some or all of these procedures are available at various medical centers, but it is not yet clear how useful each one will be. In

Table 5.1: Comparison of TNM and ABCD Staging Systems

TNM	ABCD	DESCRIPTION
T0		No evidence of tumor
T1a	A1	Clinically inapparent tumor found incidentally in tissue resected from prostate for other reasons; tumor involving 5% or less of tissue resected
T1b	A2	Clinically inapparent tumor found incidentally in tissue resected from prostate for other reasons; tumor involving more than 5% of tissue resected
T1c	B0	Tumor that cannot be felt with DRE, identified because of high PSA level in blood stream
T2a	B1	Tumor involving half (or less) of one prostate lobe
T2b	B1	Tumor involving more than half of one lobe, but not both lobes
T2c	B2	Tumor involving both lobes
T3a	C1	Unilateral extension of tumor outside prostate (one side)
T3b	C1	Bilateral extension of tumor outside prostate (both sides)
T3c	C1	Tumor invading one or both seminal vesicles
T4a	C2	Tumor invading bladder neck and/or external sphincter and/or rectum
T4b	C2	Tumor invading additional areas adjacent to prostate
N0		No regional lymph node metastasis
N1	D1	Metastasis in a single lymph node, 2 cm or less at greatest dimension
N2	D1	Metastasis in a single lymph node more than 2 cm, but no more than 5 cm at greatest dimension, or in multiple lymph nodes none more than 5 cm at greatest dimension
N3	D1	Metastasis in a lymph node more than 5 cm at greatest dimension
M0		No distant metastasis
M1 (M+)	D2	Distant metastasis, such as spinal column

From The Management of Localized Prostate Cancer: A Patient's Guide, *published by the American Urological Association Prostate Cancer Clinical Guidelines Panel. Used by permission.*

DNA PLOIDY ANALYSIS

One of the most difficult jobs for a pathologist is to judge how likely it is that an individual patient's cancer will spread or metastasize. *Flow cytometry* and *digital image analysis* are laboratory procedures that help answer that question.

Cells obtained by biopsy are stained with a fluorescent dye that attaches to cellular DNA. By measuring the relative degree to which the cells fluoresce (change color under special light), the pathologist can establish the number of complete sets of chromosomes the cells contain. These characteristics, which are described as *DNA ploidy,* appear to be related to the cancer's growth rate and its potential to metastasize.

At this time, flow cytometry and digital image analysis are being used by some laboratories as a routine part of a cancer workup. There is evidence that the DNA ploidy of biopsied cells indicates how well (or poorly) an individual prostate cancer is likely to respond to hormone therapy. This information can be very important to a man who is trying to decide whether to have hormone therapy or another treatment.

the meantime, one of the most important steps is to have clearly defined standards for clinical and pathological staging that are used throughout the world. Making sure that everyone's cancer is defined in the same way is the first step toward a reliable analysis of the best treatments for different types of cancers.

IN CONCLUSION

Before selecting a course of therapy, the patient needs to have a sense of the cancer's current state and its potential for future growth. Knowing the cancer's stage can help him evaluate his options. An early, nonaggressive tumor—for example, a nonpalpable stage T1a (or stage A1) with a low Gleason grade—may not require any treatment beyond so-called watchful waiting, with regular DRE and PSA tests to monitor for signs of progression. Older men may find this approach acceptable, since these tumors usually grow very slowly. However, younger men (that is, under the age of sixty) might choose a more aggressive therapy, such as radiation therapy, or surgery to remove the entire prostate.

As a rule, treatment options are different for more advanced, or higher, stages of cancer. Prostate cancer that is organ-confined can usually be treated with surgery or radiation therapy; cancer that extends into surrounding structures is often treated with combined therapy such as surgery followed by radiation, or radiation and hormone therapy. If there are metastases to distant tissues, hormone therapy is an appropriate choice.

Cancer staging information and your doctor's advice can help guide and inform your treatment decisions, but they cannot make them for you. There is no point in worrying too much about specific numbers, or in wasting time and energy comparing your numbers to those of other men with prostate cancer. What *is* useful is to have a general understanding of the classification systems and to keep track of any changes in your cancer's grade and stage over time. This knowledge can help you evaluate the various treatment options you may be offered.

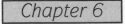

Chapter 6

Your Prostate Cancer Action Plan

A diagnosis of prostate cancer is a call to action. In this chapter we help you take full advantage of your time and resources so you can plan your next moves—moves that will determine the quality and the quantity of the rest of your life.

The strategy you devise will depend on several factors: the specific nature of your cancer; the treatment options available; the people and institutions that deliver your care; your circumstances at home and at work; and your age.

There is another factor, one that often gets overlooked when people are plunged into the chaos of dealing with a life-threatening illness. Ultimately, though, it is the most important of all: That factor is *you*. Who you are as a person will play a crucial role in shaping your course of action in the months and years ahead. To make the right choices, we recommend that you take some time to develop a solid understanding of yourself: your physical, emotional, and psychological makeup; your needs and feelings; your hopes and desires; the way you respond to challenges; your self-image as a man; your overall outlook on life.

In dealing with prostate cancer, then, it helps to

- Know your enemy: the cancer within;
- Know your allies: caregivers, family, friends;
- Know your resources: information, treatments, health care coverage, support networks;
- And know yourself: your body, mind, and spirit.

GETTING THE BIG PICTURE:
THE PHASES OF CANCER MANAGEMENT

Dealing with any form of cancer is not an event but a process. Generally, the phases and the specific tasks involved in prostate cancer are:

- Pretreatment phase
  - Getting the diagnosis
  - Discovering yourself
  - Finding your doctor(s)
  - Deciding on treatment
- Treatment phase
  - Starting treatment
  - Completing treatment
  - Dealing with immediate effects of treatment
- Posttreatment phase
  - Adjusting to life with the disease
  - Coping with fears of recurrence

If treatment does not succeed, or if the disease returns after a period of remission, the next phase and its tasks are:

- Advanced phase
  - Managing the disease
  - Considering experimental treatments
  - Preparing for death
  - Grieving
  - Adjusting to loss

In this chapter we describe the steps that every man with prostate cancer takes during the pretreatment phase. Chapters 7 through 12 cover the treatment options for prostate cancer. Chapter 13 examines the issues involved in managing advanced or recurring cancer. Chapters 14 through 16 look at the main side effects of treatment and address the need for emotional support, for both the man with prostate cancer and his partner in life.

RESPONDING TO THE DIAGNOSIS

A diagnosis of prostate cancer means facing the fact that you have a very serious but still potentially treatable disease. Following are the tasks to accomplish as you deal with your new reality.

Face the Future

Your first task is to come to grips with your mortality. It's a very human trait to believe, deep down, that you will live forever. Often it takes a shock, such as a diagnosis of cancer, to shatter that illusion. But men don't usually learn that they have prostate cancer until they are past fifty or sixty. At that point, they have accomplished many of their major goals in life. They have raised families and established careers. They have also started to sense the onset of the twilight of their years. One of the gifts of maturity is a growing sense of one's limitations. Realizing that we are allotted a certain span of years need not induce panic. Instead, it can encourage us to make the most of the time we have available to us.

Recognize and Manage Your Emotions

As you struggle to come to terms with having prostate cancer, you probably will experience a gamut of strong, often overwhelming, sometimes unfamiliar emotions. It is very common at first for men to refuse to believe they have cancer, to be afraid of what the future holds, to grieve for all they've lost or may lose, or to rage about what's happening. Often these turbulent feelings emerge in the plaintive question, "Why me?"

Many men old enough to have prostate cancer were brought up in a culture that did not encourage them to express their true

ON FEAR

Bob and I let a year go by without even talking about how scared we both were. One day we were discussing something and I just blurted out, "I'm scared to death I'll lose you." Suddenly Bob said, "I'm afraid too." That caught me off guard. I never knew he felt that way.

I think men want to take care of women and protect them, so they pretend they're not afraid. And the woman doesn't want to burden the guy by saying, "God, I'm afraid you're going to die tomorrow and I'll be left alone." So you don't discuss it. But that's not the way it should be.

If I had it to do over again, I would want to know how Bob really felt. On the second day after diagnosis, I wish I'd said, "I'm afraid, and I know you are too."

—Joan, wife of a prostate cancer survivor from California

emotions. Prostate cancer triggers anguish, fear, rage, and other powerful emotions, but some men may never have learned to recognize, let alone express, these feelings. For some men, handling emotions in an appropriate and healthy way may take some effort.

We'd like to make it clear to you and your loved ones that no response to a diagnosis of prostate cancer is "wrong." Most reactions—denial, anger, fear, shock, disbelief, regret, confusion, helplessness, panic, worry, depression, grief—are perfectly understandable and normal. Sometimes even unpleasant emotions can serve a positive purpose, motivating a person to face the tasks at hand and take action. Still, we caution you to be on the lookout for exaggerated emotional reactions—prolonged denial; debilitating depression; anger expressed in dangerous, violent, or self-destructive acts—that may be unhealthy and counterproductive.

Coping with and surviving prostate cancer will be a source of stress in the years ahead. This can be true even if your treatment results in a cure. You may pride yourself on your positive "I'm going to beat this" attitude one day, only to feel overwhelmed by fear and hopelessness the next day if your PSA level starts to rise. You need to be emotionally prepared for these moments.

A common emotion is anger. "My initial reaction was, I was really angry," recalled Virgil, age forty-nine, a sales manager from New Jersey and a Vietnam veteran. "I remember thinking, 'I don't need any more character-building at this point in my life.'"

Anger can arise in the diagnostic phase, but it may also emerge later if treatment leads to adverse effects. Many men tend to bottle up anger rather than express it constructively. Over time, unexpressed anger can turn into a deep and debilitating depression. On the other hand, some men are quick to express anger by becoming verbally abusive or physically violent. "The hard part," said Lonnie, a survivor from Kentucky, "is remembering that you're angry at the cancer—not at the people who are trying to help you get better."

Anger is not necessarily confined to the patient. As the wife of a survivor noted, "I got mad as hell because I felt the cancer was taking the man I loved away from me."

Many men with prostate cancer also feel a tremendous sense of guilt. "I tortured myself for weeks with the thought that I had done something wrong in my life, and that prostate cancer was my punishment," said Ted, a sixty-eight-year-old retired naval officer. Only after he had done his homework and found out that no one knows what causes prostate cancer or how to prevent it was Ted able to dispense with guilt and get on with the process of recovering.

Overcome Denial

A typical response to a diagnosis of prostate cancer is to deny that the problem exists. "I didn't hear anything my doctor said after he uttered the word *cancer*," recalled Parnell, a fifty-six-year-old businessman from Oregon. "Even after I saw the lab results, I chose to believe that the cancer would just go away on its own, like the flu." Parnell's attitude is a classic case of denial.

Your critical task in this phase is to move beyond denial to acceptance. Only then will you be ready to seek information about the disease, take a look at yourself and your specific needs, and make informed choices about treatment.

Assess Your Coping Strategy

Many men feel that masculinity means coping with life's problems by assuming responsibility, being in control, calling the shots. Typically men pride themselves on being strong, on providing support for others without ever showing any traces of weakness. Learning you have prostate cancer and facing your mortality may make your old, dependable coping style obsolete. It may be time to make some changes. While you cannot change how you feel, you can exert some control over how these feelings affect your life.

Whatever your reaction, always remember that you don't have to tough it out alone or in silence. Unfortunately, it is not uncommon for a man with prostate cancer to withdraw from the world. He may say that he doesn't want to be a complainer or a burden to others, and he may mean what he says. But many men withdraw because they have not had much experience recognizing or talking about their emotional needs. As a result, too many men with prostate cancer retreat behind a wall of secrecy, silence, and isolation, cut off from their loved ones, their friends, their community, even themselves.

Help is out there for you, for the asking. Virtually any health care professional you meet can provide assistance by referring you to a support group, a counselor, or other sources of assistance. Sometimes just a good talk with a doctor, friend, or loved one is all it takes. Other times you may need more. Chapter 16 discusses some of the resources available to you. The important thing is to know that you *can* reach out, and that the support you need will be there.

YOUR PATIENT PROFILE

How you respond to having cancer and how you choose which treatment depend mainly on two things: the nature of the cancer, and the nature of *you*. There are a number of factors that, taken as a whole, make up your *patient profile*.

Age

Perhaps the single most important variable, age can be measured in two distinct ways: chronologically (the number of years you've lived) and psychologically (how old you *feel*). Some men are "old" at sixty: sick, tired, ready to pack it in. Others are still "young" at eighty: active, vigorous, vital.

The younger you are chronologically, the more likely it is that surgery will be a good choice. Some research suggests that the survival benefits of surgery for early-stage cancer show up after ten or fifteen years. Put another way, the younger you are when you have surgery, the more likely it is that you'll live longer.

Some urologists refuse to do radical prostatectomies on men over a certain age, typically seventy or seventy-five. In their view, either the stress of the procedure is too great for the patient to tolerate or the benefit does not justify the treatment. But an older man in excellent health who strongly wants his early-stage tumor *gone* may do very well after prostatectomy. If you fit this description, and surgery is the only option you'll accept, you may have to look a little harder to find a doctor who will do the procedure, but eventually you will succeed.

Psychological Traits

Men handle crises, including prostate cancer, in different ways:

• Some keep problems to themselves, not wanting anyone— including their wives—to know that things are tough. Others express their feelings more readily.

• Some men want to know everything they can about a problem so they can make the right choices. Others are more passive, willing to let others make the decisions.

• Some men handle problems alone. Others seek support from outside.

• Some men can accept a certain level of uncertainty. Others demand to know precisely what is going to happen and when.

• Some men feel embarrassed talking about intimate but crucial personal problems with strangers, or even with close friends. Others are perfectly willing to speak openly and divulge intimate details of their lives.

These coping strategies are matters of personal style. One is not necessarily better than another in every case. What is important is to know which ones best describe you. Can you envision any benefit that might accrue if you were to adopt a different approach to your problems?

Sexuality

For men with prostate cancer, the issue of sex is an especially complex one. The disease tends to strike in later life, a time often marked by lower sex drive and decreased frequency of intercourse. Many healthy older men gradually lose their ability to get an erection anyway, and they have no problem adjusting.

But some men absolutely cannot think of themselves as being "a man" unless they can become erect and achieve vaginal penetration. They would rather harbor a lethal cancer than risk losing sexual function, and they won't for a minute consider hormone therapy (which often includes castration) as an option.

Sex is one of the toughest issues you'll have to wrestle with in devising your prostate cancer action plan. Ask yourself these questions:

• How important is sex to me?

• Can I accept impotence as a trade-off for the chance to live longer?

• How will I feel if I cannot achieve a natural erection? How will my partner feel?

• Am I willing to explore alternatives, such as anti-impotence drugs, a penile implant, a vacuum pump, or injections, to help obtain erections?

• Am I willing to explore other strategies for enjoying physical intimacy with my partner?

Your honest answers will have a direct bearing on the type of treatment you choose.

Emotional Makeup

In painting your patient portrait, you need to take stock of your emotional needs. Many men in our culture are not truly aware of what their feelings are, and they are uncomfortable dealing with the expression of emotions, whether their own or someone else's. For a year and a half after his prostatectomy at age sixty-one, Oscar, a prostate cancer survivor from Nebraska, was unaware that his mood was sinking lower and lower. He knew he felt sad; what he did not know was that he was caught in the grip of a true medical illness: a clinical depression. Finally he sought help from a psychiatrist, who prescribed one of the new antidepressants. "That drug saved my marriage, it saved my life—it saved *me*," he commented.

Social and Environmental Factors

How you cope with prostate cancer has a great deal to do with your situation in life. For most men, having a supportive and understanding wife or partner is the most important factor. "You have to tackle this as a team," says Larry, who with his wife, April, runs a couples' support group.

Your upbringing and medical history also play a role. If your family believed illness was a sign of weakness or shame, you will probably resist letting anyone know what you're going through. If you're used to getting medical attention, you will probably feel more comfortable talking with doctors and dealing with hospitals.

Your current family dynamics make a difference too. Those families function best who can talk openly about painful feelings, who are willing to accept help and support from others, and who are flexible enough to adapt to circumstances by adjusting family roles and rules. One important step you must take is to help your family understand your situation and help them adjust to the new situation.

Lifestyle is a big consideration. Are you active or sedentary? Working or retired? Involved in your community or isolated? Involved in hobbies and social groups or uninterested in such activities? What impact will your treatment choice have on your lifestyle?

Other factors that play a role include cultural heritage, social support, and religion.

PROSTATE CANCER AFFECTS SPOUSES, TOO

A recent survey suggests that prostate cancer can actually be more psychologically distressing for wives or partners of patients than for the men themselves. In the survey, men reported that the symptoms with the greatest impact on their lives were pain, fatigue, and increased urinary frequency. Women identified the biggest problems as their partners' lack of energy and increased urinary frequency. In grading the overall impact of these symptoms on their lives, women reported greater levels of stress than did the patients.

And partners can be affected in unexpected ways. As the wife of one of our patients put it, "If he gets up ten times a night to pee, neither one of us gets any sleep—and I don't even have a prostate!"

FINDING YOUR DOCTOR(S)

Faced with a diagnosis of prostate cancer, many men take an active role in finding the doctor they want to take care of them — and making it clear how they want to be treated. While this approach may not be right for everyone, we feel it is generally a good thing and encourage you to consider yourself as a participant in the decision-making process.

Assemble Your Team

Ideally, prostate cancer treatment involves a team of caregivers, each of whom has expertise in one of the several facets of your care. Typically, family physicians or internists are the first to suspect the presence of prostate cancer, but they do not usually initiate treatment. Instead, they will refer you to specialists who have more pertinent experience. They may also be involved in your care after your initial treatment.

In most cases you will consult a *urologist*, a physician who specializes in conditions of the genitourinary system. Some urologists even subspecialize in cancer, and most are very familiar with prostate cancer and its treatment. The urologist is usually responsible for your ongoing prostate cancer care before, during, and after treatment.

Radiation therapists are physicians who specialize in treating disease through the use of radiation. Some may even devote their practice to dealing with urologic cancers. Typically the radiation *oncologist* (cancer specialist) supervises treatment involving external-beam radiation therapy, while the actual dose is administered by a radiation *technician*. If the procedure involves seed implantation, however, the radiation oncologist — perhaps in tandem with the urologist — performs the actual procedure.

A *medical oncologist* is a physician with expertise in using chemotherapy for the treatment of cancer. Apart from hormones used in treatment, drugs are not yet available for prostate cancer (except perhaps in the advanced stages), so a medical oncologist is sel-

---

LOCATING A SPECIALIST

The easiest way to find a specialist is to ask your family doctor for a referral. Be aware, however, that some doctors will recommend someone just because they went to medical school together or because they're old friends. You can also ask family and friends, or men who have had treatment. But keep in mind that your brother-in-law's case may require a different set of medical skills than does yours. And you want the *best* doctor you can find, not merely the most *convenient* one.

Call national, state, and local medical societies or professional organizations to ask for names. (Remember, though, that these are referrals, not recommendations.) Libraries have directories of health care providers. One effective strategy is to call the urology department of a nearby hospital and ask the secretaries or nurses, "Who at your institution would *you* choose to treat your father?" The American Cancer Society is another valuable resource for help in finding a physician.

If you belong to a managed health care system, there is a strong likelihood that you will not have much say in who your specialists will be. You may also be restricted in the number of second and third opinions you can get, and, more important, in the treatment options that are available to you. And many insurance plans refuse to pay for a treatment they consider "experimental." Unfortunately, their definition of experimental can be pretty broad.

---

dom part of the team. However, some men consult with a medical oncologist to get an objective opinion from a physician who does not have a vested (or financial) interest in the treatment decision.

Verify your choice

You may need to do a little research to make sure your physician is qualified for the job. At the very least, review the doctor's credentials. Many physicians are *board-certified*, which means they have met stringent requirements (performing certain numbers and types of operations, for example) and have passed rigorous oral and written examinations. A certificate on the wall does not guarantee quality, and it is not the only measure of a good physician, but it is a strong indication that the physician has the requisite skills and experience. To find out if a doctor is board-certified, call the American Board of Medical Specialists in Chicago (1-800-776-2378).

You can also call your state board of medical examiners, which monitors complaints against physicians and keeps track of lawsuits or disciplinary actions. Remember, though, that just because a suit has been filed—or even if a settlement was reached out of court—it does not necessarily mean the doctor was guilty of malpractice. However, if the list of complaints or actions against a physician shows a pattern of repeated offenses, proceed with caution.

Ask the doctors you are considering how many prostate cancer procedures they have performed in their careers and how many they have done in the past year. This is not mere idle conversation, as Ron, a faculty dean at a New York college, discovered for himself. When he was fifty-seven, his prostate cancer was diagnosed by a urologist who told him he should have surgery within the month—surgery to be performed, of course, by that urologist. Ron decided to take more time to research the situation. Eventually he chose to have the radical prostatectomy done by an experienced surgeon in another state. "In the meanwhile," he said, "I found out my first urologist had never done a radical prostatectomy in his entire career."

Ask doctors about the outcomes: How many of their patients experience incontinence or impotence? And demand specific answers. You might hear Doctor X say, "Only five percent of my patients are permanently incontinent." Given the slippery nature of statistics, however, this remark might also mean that the other 95 percent had serious incontinence for ten years after treatment.

Another important factor in choosing a caregiver is the doctor's bedside manner. The quality of your care, and your level of satisfaction, are affected by that intangible factor called "chemistry." To feel comfortable with a caregiver, you need to take into account:

• Your personality: Are you the "give it to me straight" type or the "please be gentle" type?

• The doctor's personality: brusque and businesslike, or sensitive and sympathetic?

• The doctor's philosophy: Is it a one-treatment-fits-all approach, or does the doctor carefully weigh your individual preferences and circumstances?

• The doctor's time commitment to you: too brief, too chatty, or just right?

• Your relative ages: Are you comfortable with a doctor young enough to be your grandchild, or do you want an old-timer who's been around the block a few times (but who may not be as well versed in the latest prostate cancer research and strategies)?

Doctors are human too. The perfect physician does not exist. Decide for yourself what is most important in your relationship—personal style, professional expertise, experience—and base your choice on that.

Communicate with Your Caregivers

A number of factors can disrupt the process of communication. One critical factor is time. If a harried doctor makes you feel he doesn't have time for you, you will not feel relaxed enough to ask your questions, let alone listen to the answers.

Emotions—fear, anger, depression, even gratitude—can get in the way of your treatment. Naturally, you are afraid of the disease that is assaulting your body. But you may also be afraid to "bother" your doctor with matters that you feel may be trivial. You should always recognize your emotions and accept them as part of the process, but don't let them dominate the scene.

Many patients complain about the technical language doctors use. Sometimes a medical term is the most precise way to make our point. If you don't understand something, say so. Make the most of your time with the doctor. Prepare your list of questions in advance. Ideally, you should bring someone with you—your wife, a friend— to hear what the doctor says and to ask questions of their own.

Watch for Bias

Bias is a natural human characteristic, and doctors are only human. As one prostate cancer survivor put it, "You can't ask Cadillac salesmen what they think of the BMW and expect an objective answer." A study published in 1988 found that, sure enough, urologists would overwhelmingly choose radical prostatectomy as their treatment if they had prostate cancer, while radiation oncologists would overwhelmingly choose radiation therapy. (Medical oncologists split the ticket.) Your doctors should be forthcoming about any biases. If they don't bring up the topic, you should. This becomes especially important if you choose not to follow their recommendation. You may feel guilty for going against their advice, or feel that you are disappointing or insulting them. Remember, it's your body and your life. Do not be passive or too dependent on someone else for decisions that should ultimately be your own.

Consider Getting a Second Opinion

Doctors themselves frequently consult with other experts to make sure they're on the right track. Pathologists, for example, often ask colleagues to look at a tissue sample and give their opinion. Some insurers even *require* you to get a second opinion. If you are unsure about what course to follow, consider obtaining a second opinion.

Here are a few guidelines for getting a different perspective:

• Talk to doctors in different specialties.

• Go outside your doctor's practice. Two doctors who share an office may be reluctant to contradict each other.

• If your prostate cancer is in an advanced stage, talk to a medical oncologist.

• If your insurer won't cover the cost of a second opinion, try to find a way to pay for it yourself. It can be that important.

• Take charge of seeing that your medical records are available to the second physician before your appointment.

• If possible, bring your wife, partner, or a friend along.

• It is acceptable to change doctors, but don't change just because you're hoping to hear a more positive assessment of your illness. And excessive "doctor-shopping" can delay treatment and be confusing and harmful.

DECIDING ON TREATMENT

Prostate cancer poses tough choices. Depending on your test results, you will have to choose whether to wait and see what happens, to undergo an operation, to have radiation treatments, or to do something else entirely. Only you can decide which of many potentially difficult side effects you would be willing to live with, and whether you are more concerned about the quantity of your life or its quality.

Study your options

Prostate cancer survivors often complain that doctors did not tell them what all of their options were. Realistically, though, not all options are available for all men at all stages of the disease. And some treatments have not proved to be of much value. Generally, the earlier the stage, the more choices you have (see box).

Keep in mind that your first shot at treatment is your best. It may not always be possible to try another approach if the first one does not work. Approach your first treatment decision as if it is the only one you will make.

How do you make a choice?

One good way is to become informed. Many men want to learn everything they can about their disease and its treatment. They read voraciously, get second opinions, talk to other men, join support groups, and go online.

That's fine, but here are some caveats:

It may not be possible to acquire and absorb all the information in the relatively short time available before you have to "choose your weapon" against prostate cancer. The information may not present a clear, consistent picture. Second opinions often contradict first opinions. Articles and books may reflect a deep bias. The prostate cancer survivors you meet may insist that the choice they made is the right one for everybody. Remember, though, that everyone's case is unique. Just because one man had a great (or terrible) experience with a certain therapy or doctor does not mean you will have a similar outcome.

Finally, our advice is to do your fact-finding *before* you decide on a treatment. And resist the temptation to make your choice and then look for a doctor to carry out your plan.

Talk to your doctors. They can provide reliable information. Often they can provide you with copies of medical articles, patient literature, or other useful materials.

Another good source of input is a support group. Many people assume, incorrectly, that such groups are only open to people after they have had treatment. But if you are newly diagnosed, you may find it enormously helpful to meet with, and ask questions of, other men who collectively have "seen it all." Ideally, the group will be one that allows wives and partners to participate or that has a spouse's group, because no doubt your wife or partner has many questions, too.

TREATMENT OPTIONS BY STAGE

• Stage T1a cancers may be small and are not immediately life-threatening. Many men will do well with watchful waiting.

• Stage T1b, T1c, and T2 cancers are usually larger or more aggressive. Watchful waiting may be an option, but usually more decisive treatment is called for. Surgery, radiation, hormone therapy, or other approaches can be considered.

• Stage T3 cancers are usually treated with surgery or radiation. In some cases, a combination of surgery and radiation may be tried. Some patients do well taking hormones to shrink the tumor prior to surgery or radiation.

• Stages N+ and M+ cancers—cancers that have spread—usually involve hormone therapy or radiation therapy to slow down the progression of the disease. Some men may opt for watchful waiting combined with palliative treatment to address symptoms should they occur. Surgery coupled with hormone therapy may be useful in patients with microscopic lymph node metastases.

If you are computer literate, you can find a lot of material online. The American Cancer Society has a large site on the World Wide Web (http://www.cancer.org). Several other helpful websites are available, some dealing specifically with prostate cancer. See the resources section at the back of this book for suggestions.

Computer bulletin boards are great for exchanging personal anecdotes and information, but you should always be on guard for overly optimistic accounts of "miracle" treatments that have not undergone rigorous clinical testing. Be aware of marketing claims that play on your emotions but lack substance. Misinformation can come from any direction, and you don't know for certain who's sitting in front of the computer on the other end. Whenever you do online research, consider the source of the information before accepting it as accurate or true.

For some reason, when certain people find out you have cancer, they just can't wait to tell you their own stories. Try to remain compassionate during these tales of woe; these people are struggling with their own fears about cancer.

Some men study the disease so much and for so long that they develop "analysis paralysis." Unable to make sense of confusing, conflicting statistics and mind-numbing technical terms, they lose their way. On the other hand, some men read an article or two, or watch a TV show about prostate cancer, and decide that's enough. The best approach lies somewhere between these two extremes.

Give yourself a reasonable amount of time—say, two hours a day over two or three weeks—to research the subject. After that period, choose a treatment. Then take another week to mull over your decision. If you don't feel comfortable, you have some more soul-searching to do. Meanwhile, you may want to ask your doctor about hormone therapy, which can slow down the progression of your cancer and buy you some more time—perhaps three months, perhaps even a year—for deciding on a more aggressive, cure-attempting strategy. (Remember, though, that hormone therapy is not without side effects, nor can it guarantee that the cancer will not progress.)

Know the Risks

No one can predict what problems, if any, you will experience after treatment. But, as Jim Mullen of Man to Man puts it, "Do the research, then decide on the worst-case scenario that you feel you can live with."

Build Your Support Network

The pretreatment phase is the best time to begin developing a network of people and services that can provide the practical, emotional, and social support you will need in the years to come.

The most important support system, of course, is your family.

Over the years, you and your wife or partner, your children, and the members of your extended family have developed patterns of communicating and interacting. The diagnosis of a serious illness will test the strength of those patterns. If, for example, you are not used to speaking openly about health issues, your natural response will be to keep your prostate cancer to yourself. However, if your family holds regular meetings to discuss issues, then no doubt this item will appear at the top of your agenda.

Openness and honesty will serve you better in the long run than will secrecy. Let your loved ones know what you're dealing with. Share what you've learned, ask for their thoughts, and listen to their input. Prepare to reorganize the family structure to accommodate the new circumstances. For example, you might want to nominate one family member to be the "point person," handling calls from concerned relatives and passing along status reports when needed.

Friends are another important element of your network. Many men limit their discussions with their buddies to "safe" topics: sports, golf, cars, the weather. You need to determine whether your friends would rather *not* know about your crisis—indeed, if they may even avoid you if they know you're sick and suffering—or whether they will stand by you. In times of crisis, people can feel let down by someone they always assumed would "be there" for them. If that happens to you, it can be painful. Remind yourself that such a person is not rejecting you; instead, he is wrestling with his own fears about illness and mortality. On the other hand, crises often bring out the best in others. People in need are often pleasantly surprised to discover how much others do care about them.

Members of the clergy can also play a key role. Spiritual counselors can help you come to grips with mortality, set priorities, and face up to important decisions. It's normal for men to want such guidance when wrestling with life-and-death issues.

Your hospital or care center can put you in touch with people who are skilled at addressing emotional and practical issues. Counselors can work with you on marital or personal problems; therapists can help you overcome depression and anxiety; social workers can locate sources of financial aid or home health care.

And support groups can provide information, guidance, understanding . . . even love. Attend a meeting and you will see that you don't have to go through this alone.

Make Your Decision

You can read every word ever written on prostate cancer, and talk to every man who has ever had the disease, and get opinions from every doctor in the world. At some point, though, the time will arrive when you, and you alone, must decide what to do. Ask yourself:

· Do I want to live as long as possible, or do I want to live only as long as I am in full control of my body?

· Can I accept having cancer inside my body, or do I want to do whatever it takes to have that cancer removed?

· Am I prepared for the follow-up process—doctor visits, blood tests, biopsies, scans, medications, and more procedures?

· Have I considered all the possible risks each treatment option carries?

· What does being a man mean to me? If I can't have an erection or if I lose my testicles, will I still consider myself a man?

· Will I do anything I can to get my erections back, or am I willing to learn new ways to become intimate with my partner?

· How will I deal with the impact of incontinence on my way of life?

• Have I taken into account the feelings of my wife or partner and family?

• If I knew I would die tomorrow, how would I want to live today?

Once you have made your choice, and feel comfortable with it, the time to act is at hand.

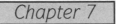

Watchful Waiting

If you have been told you have early-stage prostate cancer, you are wrestling with a series of difficult, life-affecting questions:

- Which treatment is best for me?

- Which has the fewest side effects?

- Which side effects can I live with most easily?

Another important question is, *When—if ever—do I need to get treatment?*

That this question can even arise is due to the fact that, compared to other cancers, prostate cancer grows slowly. When the tumor stays within the gland, two years or more may elapse before it doubles in size. In some cases, the cancer never spreads beyond the prostate at all. Prostate cancer that is diagnosed early and is not especially aggressive may give you time to evaluate your options and make the treatment decision that's best for you.

If you absolutely, positively knew that the cancer had not spread beyond the prostate and that the tumor was likely to grow slowly and never to spread, you would want to think long and hard before undergoing any treatment (such as radiation or surgery) that might cause serious adverse effects (such as incontinence or impotence) without necessarily adding years to your life.

On the other hand, if you absolutely, positively knew that your cancer was the aggressive type that might one day spread, causing pain and suffering and shortening your life, you would probably be inclined to take steps as soon as possible to eliminate or at least halt the progression of your disease.

Watchful waiting is what you do until you find out which category fits your situation.

CONFUSION ABOUNDS

Today, roughly one man in three with prostate cancer is treated with some form of watchful waiting at some point. In reading about the subject, you'll run across such related phrases as "expectant management," "active surveillance," "conservative therapy," "observation and follow-up," "posttreatment monitoring," and even "delayed treatment." We generally prefer "expectant management," but since "watchful waiting" is the term most widely used both by physicians and men with prostate cancer, we'll use it—albeit with some reluctance—in this book.

To add to the confusion, there is no single, official textbook definition of what "watchful waiting" actually means. With some doctors, it can indicate that you will receive no treatment whatsoever. With others, it may mean you have received treatment and are now being monitored to see if the treatment worked. Everything depends on a wide range of factors, including your age and general health, results of tests you have undergone to date, your personal attitude, and the experience and expertise of the doctor handling your case.

WATCHFUL WAITING IS *NOT* "DOING NOTHING"

The phrase "watchful waiting" is misleading, because it suggests that this is a very passive approach. That is not the case. Keeping watch over your cancer can be a highly active process—as active as you and your doctor deem necessary to put you in the best position to meet your treatment objectives.

Nor does choosing watchful waiting mean you are avoiding making a decision. On the contrary, it means you must aggressively develop a range of options for yourself.

EARLY-STAGE PROSTATE CANCER *GIVES* YOU TIME; WATCHFUL WAITING *BUYS* YOU TIME

In recent years, more and more men have been choosing one of the watchful waiting options described below. The primary reason for this trend is that improved screening and earlier diagnosis mean more cancers are being found in younger men and at earlier stages, which may allow more time to consider options.

Because prostate cancer grows slowly, it is possible to think of the disease as a chronic condition that must be *managed* as long as possible. Managing means keeping close tabs on the cancer's status and making contingency plans for what to do if and when it gets worse.

Prostate cancer is most treatable when it is still confined to the prostate gland. Unfortunately, there is simply no way to predict if untreated cancer will spread, or when, or how fast.

Research is under way to determine if prostate cancer cells carry telltale clues revealing whether they will progress and become a threat or remain latent and basically harmless. If we could peer into the microscope, analyze a cell's "personality," and predict its future, we could then suggest with confidence that men with prostate cancer consider watchful waiting. Such a development, however, is not likely to occur anytime soon.

REASONS FOR WATCHFUL WAITING

There are at least three approaches to treatment that involve watchful waiting at some point in the process.

Cure-Delaying Watchful Waiting

The goal of this strategy is to try for a cure with definitive treatment after a period of watchful waiting. You and your doctor carefully weigh all the factors in your case—stage and grade of the cancer, pattern of PSA levels over a period of time, your personal circumstances and preferences, and so on. You then decide that you'll undergo aggressive treatment aimed at eliminating the cancer, with the understanding that you will defer that therapy until some diagnostic landmark has been reached, such as a specific rise in PSA level. Your doctor then monitors your disease carefully. As soon as signs indicate that the cancer is advancing—even if you are not experiencing symptoms—the treatment you've selected will begin.

A typical candidate for this approach is a man in his late sixties to early seventies who has an early-stage localized cancer and whose PSA has been steady for several years (see Table 7.1). Given the slow rate at which many prostate cancers grow, this man stands a good chance of dying from some other cause before the prostate cancer becomes life-threatening. Should the cancer progress, however, he may still be a candidate for surgery, radiation, or hormone therapy. Typically, the man who chooses this approach has concluded that he would rather live with the knowledge he has prostate cancer and risk more extensive and serious illness later than suffer the side effects of treatment today.

Some caveats are in order. Before choosing this form of management, a man must fully understand that clinical estimates of the aggressiveness and extent of prostate cancer are often inaccurate, and commonly underestimate the true status of the cancer. It is entirely possible that after a period of several years of watchful waiting, the disease will ultimately prove to be incurable when a decision finally is made to attempt a cure. Furthermore, other medical problems may arise during this watchful waiting period (such as a heart attack or stroke) that would preclude aggressive curative surgical measures. Clearly, cure-delaying watchful waiting may entail significant risks.

TABLE 7.1: CANDIDATES FOR WATCHFUL WAITING	
WATCHFUL WAITING APPROACH	**INDICATION**
Delaying treatment	• Cancer is localized and well or moderately differentiated (Gleason score 6 or less) • Cancer is newly diagnosed, Stage T1 or T2 • Patient is in early 70s or older • Patient has decided to undergo treatment when signs indicate that cancer has progressed
Posttreatment; combination (intermittent)	• Patient has undergone primary therapy (prostatectomy; radiation) • PSA levels are low and stable
Managing symptoms	• Prostate cancer is too advanced for hope of curative therapy • Patient's health is too frail to withstand surgery or radiation • Expected life span is less than 5–10 years • Cancer is Stage T3, N+, or M+ but no symptoms are present

Most of the discussion in this chapter is aimed at this category of watchfully waiting patient, the one who has opted to go for the cure when the time is right. To keep things simple, the term "watchful waiting" will generally refer to this treatment-delaying strategy. When necessary, we will distinguish between this approach and the other strategies outlined next.

Posttreatment Watchful Waiting

Even after curative therapy, there is often a significant chance that prostate cancer can recur. A single cancer cell can escape initial treatment and hide somewhere in the body, proliferating for years until it advances enough to produce a new, detectable tumor. That is why you need to stay constantly vigilant even after radical prostatectomy or intensive radiation therapy.

In the strategy we'll call *posttreatment watchful waiting*, a man undergoes a primary course of therapy, then returns to his doctor for regular PSA tests and perhaps repeat biopsies. If these tests indicate the return or progression of cancer, his main option is to begin hormone therapy to arrest or slow down the progression of the disease. In a few cases, additional aggressive therapies may be tried, such as repeating the initial therapy (in the case of, say, cryosurgery) or "salvage" treatment (such as radical prostatectomy following radiation treatment).

Symptom-Managing Watchful Waiting

After weighing the evidence, and taking careful stock of your needs and desires, you and your doctors may conclude that curative treatment will not result in enhancement of either the quality or the quantity of your life. In such circumstances, you may choose not to undergo therapy, opting instead to keep alert for signs the cancer is progressing. If and when symptoms arise that cause pain or discomfort, they will be treated. But with the symptom-managing watchful waiting (some experts call this "pure" watchful waiting), a man essentially decides in advance that no real attempt will be made to cure the disease, either now or later. The goal here is to live with the cancer and deal with its consequences for as long and as painlessly as possible.

Good candidates for this approach include men in their late seventies or eighties whose prostate cancer is low Gleason grade with stable PSA level and negative bone scans. Men who suffer from other serious health problems or who have a life expectancy less than ten years might also consider this strategy, and it would also be appropriate for a man who is younger but whose general health is such that he is unable to endure the physical strain of surgery or radiation. Symptom-managing watchful waiting may also be appropriate for some men whose cancer is diagnosed at an advanced stage (N+) but is not causing symptoms.

WHAT TO DO WHILE YOU'RE WAITING

Take Stock of Yourself

The period immediately following your diagnosis is a time to get to know yourself better. The type of person you are will affect the type of treatment that makes the most sense for you. You may also consider taking personal stock again if and when your situation changes. Watchful waiting can span many years; circumstances—and people—can change in that time.

Stay in Touch with Your Caregivers

Don't think that watchful waiting means you'll never have to visit a doctor or endure another DRE again. With watchful waiting, you may actually spend *more* time dealing with doctors and the health care system than you would with some other strategies.

Although every case is different, your doctor will probably recommend that you have a PSA test and a DRE at least several times a year. If your PSA remains stable, you may be able to reduce the number of these tests, but if you are particularly anxious about your condition, you may want to undergo them more often.

As technology improves, many doctors are increasingly using transrectal ultrasound (TRUS) to monitor their watchful waiting patients.

Consider Hormones

Many experts today advocate that patients use combination hormone therapy while in watchful waiting. Hormones can slow down the progression of the disease and buy you even more time for making an informed decision.

Among the drawbacks of hormone therapy are side effects such as hot flashes, mood changes, and loss of libido. There is also a risk that, over time—sometimes within as little as sixty to ninety days—your tumor may become *refractory*, or unresponsive to the hormones. Sometimes if you stop taking hormones for a while, they may become effective again later.

Deal with Symptoms

If you begin to experience symptoms that cause pain or discomfort, you will need to take steps to find relief. Urinary problems such as difficulty voiding, small stream, frequency, or urgency might be helped by *transurethral resection of the prostate (TURP)*, popularly known as the "Roto-Rooter" operation. An instrument known as a *resectoscope* is inserted through the penis into the prostatic urethra. The lens and the viewing system on the scope allow the physician to see into the prostate and chip away prostate tissue in tiny fragments, which are then removed through the tube. The procedure is often used to treat benign prostatic hyperplasia (BPH) and is very effective at relieving pressure on the urethra. Within three to six weeks, most men have recovered fully and are able to once again urinate without difficulty. While TURP provides symptomatic relief, it is not a cure for cancer.

You may have to undergo additional scans to check for metastases to other tissues or bone. If the cancer does spread, radiation therapy and medications can provide relief from pain. Treatment may also include hormone therapy or orchiectomy (removal of the testicles) to slow the advance of a growing cancer.

Prepare for the Worst by Living Your Best

For some men, watchful waiting also offers an opportunity to re-order their priorities in life. "Prostate cancer is the first serious disease I've ever dealt with," observes Terry, a fifty-three-year-old insurance claims adjuster from Missouri. "When it hit me that I probably wouldn't live forever, I realized I was missing out on some of the better things in my life. Lately my wife and I have started square dancing, I take more afternoons off to enjoy walks in the country, and I'm spending more time with friends. I chose to 'do nothing'—but in reality I've never been more active. I want to make sure I'm putting more life in my years, even if there may be fewer years in my life."

Many men also find peace of mind by making sure that all of their financial affairs have been settled, so that their families won't suffer unduly if death should come.

WHEN IS IT TIME FOR TREATMENT?

An elevated PSA level or an increase found in two or three tests within two to three months strongly suggests renewed growth of the cancer. PSA levels of 10.0 ng/mL or higher may signal that the cancer is spreading outside of the prostate. While in some men this may indicate that it is too late to attempt curative treatment, in other cases it could be the sign that it is time to exit the watchful waiting mode and go for treatment. Your doctor might order an ultrasound to get a good look at the prostate, or a repeat bone scan to see if there are any "hot spots" to indicate metastases.

Of course, if you a notice a change in urinary habits, or experience fatigue, weight loss, or bone pain, let your doctor know immediately.

MAKING—AND LIVING WITH—THE CHOICE

Morty is a seventy-four-year-old retired magazine editor whose prostate cancer was diagnosed two years ago. His PSA at diagnosis was 11 ng/mL and it has stayed there, plus or minus a point, for the past year. His DRE is normal, he has no symptoms, and his scans are clean. "After my initial diagnosis, I consulted a slew of urologists and radiation specialists," he says. "They all told me I should get carved or get zapped. But I decided instead just to keep an eye on things. Since then, I've been in good health. I sleep through the night without having to get up to pee. I still enjoy the good life, sexually, emotionally, and in every other way. In fact, my life is even better, because I've become vividly aware of how precious each day is."

Fred, a retired Air Force officer now living in Florida, hasn't been so lucky. When his early cancer was diagnosed at age sixty-eight, he decided to take his chances and wait for the right moment to attempt a cure. Three years later, with a rising PSA and a biopsy showing that his Gleason score had risen from 6 to 7, he underwent radiation seed–implant therapy. Over the next two years, he developed serious heart disease and had a triple bypass operation, from which he was slow to recover. Not long afterward, tests showed that the radiation had come too late; some cancer cells had escaped from the prostate and had metastasized. Because of his overall health, Fred and his doctors decided he couldn't withstand the stress of "salvage" surgery to remove his prostate. In an effort to control the progression of the disease, Fred underwent castration and is taking hormones. He also takes medications to relieve his pain and an antidepressant to help him deal with feelings of extreme sadness and helplessness.

TO WAIT OR NOT TO WAIT?

The debate over watchful waiting goes something like this: *Am I willing to risk some quantity of life in return for the assurance of continued quality of life—at least over the short term?* The watchful waiting candidate answers that question with a cautious yes.

Men and their physicians cite a range of reasons for and against the watchful waiting approach. Here are some of the main points in the discussion. You need to determine for yourself whether these are persuasive for you—one way or the other.

WATCHFUL WAITING: THE PROS AND CONS

Watchful Waiting: The Pros

LACK OF CONCLUSIVE EVIDENCE ABOUT TREATMENTS

After reviewing the available prostate cancer statistics, some men conclude that the scientific evidence does not demonstrate with absolute certainty which treatment for localized prostate cancer is best. For example, many studies indicate that radical prostatectomy and radiation therapy can be equally effective. And we don't yet have enough long-term data to indicate which of the experimental treatments, if any, enhance survival. Further muddying the waters, some research indicates that, for older men with early localized cancer, none of the available treatments appears to extend life by a significant amount. In a few years, long-term studies now under way may help us resolve these issues.

NO IMMEDIATE ADVERSE EFFECTS

Cure-attempting treatment for prostate cancer can lead to incontinence and impotence. Men can learn to accept, manage, and even overcome these inconveniences and indignities (see chapters 14 and 15), but if they can be avoided altogether, so much the better. For some men, the choice of watchful waiting means that prostate cancer will produce only minimal impact on their lives and their lifestyles.

LOW INITIAL COST

Watchful waiting is the least expensive treatment alternative, at least in the short run. However, if a cure is attempted later, or if additional treatments are needed because a therapy failed or because the stage and grade of the cancer were more aggressive than first believed, treatment becomes more complicated and the costs can rise significantly.

SAME CHOICES MAY BE AVAILABLE LATER

For those who select cure-delaying watchful waiting, it helps to know that treatment choices may be the same later—basically, radical prostatectomy or radiation—as they would have been had they undergone therapy at the outset. For many men, choosing watchful waiting does not necessarily limit the options available in the future.

HOPE FOR BETTER THINGS

In a few cases, a man chooses watchful waiting in hopes that the near future will bring some new discovery that increases the chances of a cure. Such a strategy might be better named "wishful waiting."

Watchful Waiting: The Cons

MISSED OPPORTUNITY FOR A CURE

Early-stage prostate cancer offers a "window of curability"—a period of time when a patient has his best chance of being cured. The main trouble with watchful waiting is that it gives the cancer a chance to grow and spread beyond the prostate. If a man waits too long, the window of curability may shut forever. If you and your caregivers misjudge the situation—for example, if the tumor was assigned too low a stage or grade—you will have fewer options available for managing the illness, and some of those options pose serious risks. Among our patients who chose waiting rather than treatment for their early-stage cancer, many have expressed regret at having missed the opportunity for a cure.

CLOUDY CRYSTAL BALL

With watchful waiting, you're essentially betting that you have some time before the cancer poses a threat. You're counting on frequent checkups to alert you early on to any significant changes. If you're in your late seventies or early eighties, you're assuming you will probably die of something else—and there's an excellent chance that you're right.

But here's the rub: If you live longer than you expected, or if your cancer advances faster than you predicted, you might need to undergo more aggressive treatments or procedures. By then, the best time for effective treatment may have passed.

PSA IS NOT A PERFECT PREDICTOR

Watchful waiting involves watching for a rise in your PSA level. Generally, if your PSA level is 4.0 ng/mL or less, you're in the best position to attempt a cure. As your PSA level rises, so do the odds that the cancer has begun spreading outside the wall of the prostate. But PSA levels give only an indirect idea of what the prostate cancer is up to. No one can predict with certainty at what point prostate cancer will cross the border between curable and incurable. Even if you religiously get regular PSA tests, you may be one of the 25 percent of men—one out of four—whose prostate cancer grows without producing an early-warning rise in PSA level. Waiting until there is unambiguous evidence that cancer is progressing may mean you have waited too long.

FEWER OPTIONS

Should the cancer spread beyond the prostate during the watchful waiting period, total cure is no longer an option. The strategy then shifts to slowing down the spread of the cancer, often through hormone or radiation therapy.

ANXIETY

If you're the type of man who will feel terribly anxious about harboring a malignant, unpredictable, and potentially lethal disease in your body, watchful waiting may lead to a high level of stress for both yourself and your loved ones.

RISK OF INCREASED COST

Treatment that begins only after the cancer has spread is more complicated and unlikely to result in cure. The cost, both financially *and emotionally*, can be higher.

As you can see, watchful waiting is a difficult balancing act. Your medical team can give you lots of advice on the medical pros and cons. Other prostate cancer survivors can tell you about their experiences. Counselors and others in the helping professions can teach you effective coping strategies. But in the final analysis, the person who has to make this decision—and live with it—is you.

HOW EFFECTIVE IS WATCHFUL WAITING?

Today, a number of cancer experts are recommending watchful waiting as a reasonable alternative to conventional treatments for a carefully selected group of patients. Results of recent scientific tests support their view.

Several studies report that treating localized prostate cancer with surgery or radiation has not been proved to work any better than watchful waiting. Keep in mind, however, that simply saying something has not been proved does not mean that its opposite *has* been proved. Whether early treatment is beneficial is still a subject of debate.

In contrast, it has been shown that countries where watchful waiting is the preferred approach have the highest death rates from prostate cancer. Examples include Sweden, Finland, and the United Kingdom. Still, a 1992 Swedish study that tracked 223 older men with early prostate cancer found that after 10 years, only 19 of them (8.5 percent) had died from prostate cancer, while 105 (nearly half) had died from other causes. (The rest were still alive; it remains to be seen how often prostate cancer

THE NUMBERS GAME

The Patient Outcomes Research Team (PORT), a federally funded research group, recently analyzed data from a number of prostate cancer studies. From this work—known as a meta-analysis—PORT developed a computer model that estimates life expectancy following treatment for prostate cancer. The researchers found no evidence that early treatment improved the outcome for most cancer patients. According to PORT, a sixty-year-old man with moderately aggressive cancer who opts for watchful waiting might expect to live another sixteen years, while a sixty-year-old who undergoes either radical prostatectomy or radiation therapy might expect to live seventeen years. The benefit is calculated to be even less as age advances. A study published in the *Journal of the American Medical Association* in 1993, for example, concluded that a sixty-five-year-old man treated with radical prostatectomy might live only a few weeks longer than he would have without aggressive therapy.

PORT researchers also observed that "invasive treatment generally appears to be harmful for patients older than 70 years." Above age 75, they further concluded, men "are not likely to benefit from either radiation therapy or radical prostatectomy when compared with watchful waiting."

The PORT findings have not gone unchallenged. Other investigators have found serious flaws of one kind or another in many of the studies included in PORT's meta-analysis. Further research is needed before we have more definitive answers.

will turn out to be the cause of death in this group.) Other experts have challenged these studies on the grounds of selection bias—that is, the way researchers chose which patients to include may have influenced results. But the results do tend to confirm the notion that men are more likely to die *with* prostate cancer than *from* it.

On the surface, there would appear to be strong arguments in favor of watchful waiting. Unfortunately, many of the studies that have been done have serious flaws. The methods used to gather data, the quality of the results, and the lack of control groups have cast considerable doubt on some of the findings. In fact, experts have raised objections to just about every study that has tried to analyze the effectiveness of various prostate cancer treatments.

That situation should change, and soon. Better-designed, more comprehensive studies are under way right now. But the same slowness of prostate cancer growth that makes watchful waiting an option also means that a decade or longer must elapse before the success of a particular treatment is known. One ongoing research project, known as the Prostate Cancer Intervention Versus Observation Trial (PIVOT) study, will follow 2,000 men over a 15-year period. Researchers hope to establish once and for all whether early treatment with radical prostatectomy produces better results than watchful waiting. Results won't be known until early in the next century. Until then, your best sources of up-to-the-minute information on watchful waiting are your medical team, professional organizations such as the American Cancer Society, and the various prostate cancer support groups.

THE BOTTOM LINE

Watchful waiting is an accepted method of managing prostate cancer. Far from being a "hands-off" approach, watchful waiting calls on you to decide *whether* you will undergo aggressive treatment at a later time, *what* that treatment will be, and *when* it will start. During watchful waiting, you carefully monitor your condition, watching for signs that the cancer is progressing. Many men on watchful waiting also take hormones to control their cancer and give them additional time, and you may want to do so too.

You may want to consider watchful waiting if:

- You are at least seventy years old
- Your prostate cancer is diagnosed at an early stage

- Your cancer has a low Gleason score
- You can deal with the anxiety of living with cancer inside you
- You do not want to incur the risk of side effects from treatment
- You suffer from other health problems

You probably are *not* a candidate for watchful waiting if:

- You are under seventy years of age
- You are otherwise healthy
- Your cancer has a high Gleason score
- You would be more comfortable if you undertook potentially curative therapy sooner rather than later

Chapter 8

Surgery

Whenever possible, doctors try to cure prostate cancer by permanently removing or destroying all cancerous tissue. If *curative treatment* is not an option—if, for example, the tumor has grown beyond the prostate or has metastasized—then *palliative treatment* is offered to relieve symptoms.

The two main forms of curative treatment are surgery and radiation. In this chapter we'll discuss how surgery is performed, what to expect during the operation, and how to decide whether surgery is the right choice for you.

THE SURGICAL SOLUTION

The procedure for removing a cancerous prostate gland is *radical prostatectomy*. The word *radical* here should not be frightening: It simply means getting to the *root* of the problem; in this case, by removing the entire prostate (Fig. 8.1).

To improve the odds of success, a border, or margin, of tissue surrounding the diseased prostate is also removed. If under the microscope this margin is negative (that is, free of cancer), then there's a good chance the surgery "got it all." Achieving negative surgical margins means some of the delicate muscles that help provide urinary control and some or all of the nerves that produce erections may be injured. If surgery does not remove every cancerous cell, there is a risk that the cancer will continue to develop and spread.

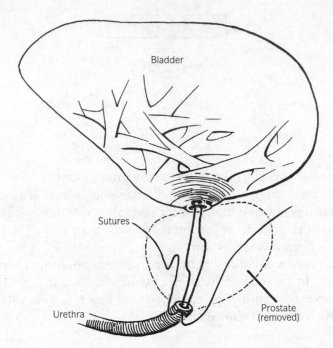

Figure 8.1: Tissue removed during radical prostatectomy.

DIFFERENT TYPES OF RADICAL PROSTATECTOMY

There are three main ways to perform the radical prostatectomy, depending on the direction from which the surgeon approaches and the extent of the nerve-sparing effort (Fig. 8.2).

In the *radical retropubic prostatectomy,* an incision is made in the lower abdomen. Before removing the prostate, the surgeon may take out the pelvic lymph nodes located on either side of the gland. If your PSA level and Gleason score are very low, and if the amount of cancer found after the biopsy is small, your surgeon may decide to leave your lymph nodes intact because the possibility that the cancer has spread outside of the

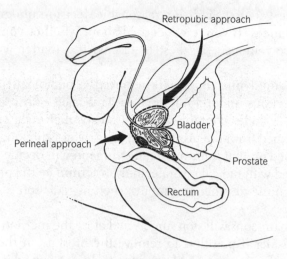

Figure 8.2: Different approaches to performing radical prostatectomy.

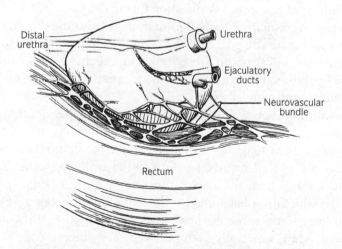

Figure 8.3: Diagram of the prostate indicating how the neurovascular bundles are connected.

prostate is very low. This is a reasonable decision under certain circumstances. If you're concerned about whether your lymph nodes are removed, it's best to discuss the matter with your surgeon.

When the lymph nodes are removed, a pathologist analyzes frozen sections under a microscope. This takes only a few minutes. If the nodes contain cancer, it means that malignant cells have escaped from the prostate and the cancer is no longer localized. Based on that information, the surgeon will decide whether to proceed with radical prostatectomy or terminate the procedure and recommend other treatments, such as radiation therapy or hormones.

Some surgeons will stop surgery and close the incision because they consider it pointless to remove the prostate in the face of lymph node metastases. Many doctors do not consider surgical excision a cure for nonlocalized prostate cancer. However, other surgeons believe that removing the entire prostate and reducing tumor size (*debulking* the tumor) is beneficial even after cancer has reached the lymph nodes, especially when surgery is followed by adjuvant hormonal or radiation therapy.

The *nerve-sparing radical prostatectomy* also uses the retropubic approach. The goal here is to preserve, to the extent possible, the nerves and structures responsible for erection. To accomplish this operation, the surgeon must have expert knowledge of pelvic anatomy and exquisite skill.

Naturally, you would want to have your erectile nerves spared if you possibly could. However, if the cancer has spread to the nerves or their neighboring blood vessels (the *neurovascular bundle*)—a fact that cannot be determined until the procedure is under way—then the nerves must be taken out (Figs. 8.3 and 8.4). If the tumor has spread to the nerves on only one side of the prostate, some surgeons leave the nerves on the other side in place. Men, especially younger men, can have erections even with just one intact bundle.

Other surgeons are unwilling to leave behind any tissue that

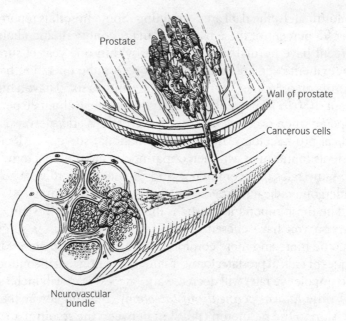

Prostate

Wall of prostate

Cancerous cells

Neurovascular
bundle

*Figure 8.4: Cancer cells migrating from the prostate
into the adjacent nerves and blood vessels.*

may be harboring cancerous cells. They assume that if cancer has
affected one set of nerves, it may also have affected the other, so
they will play it safe by removing both sides.

Nerve-sparing surgery is usually reserved for men with localized prostate cancer who undergo retropubic prostatectomy.
The final decision to attempt the procedure must be made after
the operation has begun and the surgeon has a clear view of the
prostate and adjoining nerve bundles, and after it has been established that the cancer has not spread. Therefore, it would not
be prudent for a surgeon to make any guarantees prior to
surgery.

What are the odds that nerve-sparing radical prostatectomy will
cure your cancer, preserve erections, and minimize incontinence?

Unfortunately, the data are conflicting. Some hospitals report that over 95 percent of these patients remain continent and about 70 percent have normal sexual relations within one year of surgery. The patient's age and potency status before the operation have a bearing on outcome. Younger men (age fifty to sixty) have a higher chance (50 to 70 percent) of preserving potency; about 20 percent of potent men over seventy can have erections after nerve-sparing radical prostatectomy. In contrast, a national survey of Medicare patients found men with nerve-sparing radical prostatectomy had the same rates of incontinence and impotence as those who had undergone radical prostatectomy without nerve sparing.

The most important statistic is the success rate of the particular surgeon you have chosen. To find out, simply ask. As surgeons become more and more comfortable performing the newest techniques of radical prostatectomy, it stands to reason that incontinence and impotence rates will decrease and success rates will increase.

In the *radical perineal prostatectomy*, the surgeon makes an incision in the perineum (the skin between the scrotum and the anus). This approach can require less operating time and therefore reduces the length of time the patient spends under anesthesia, making it a better choice for men who have heart or lung problems. However, it is not usually recommended for men with larger tumors. One drawback to this approach is that the surgeon does not have access to pelvic lymph nodes. To get around that problem, some doctors first do a separate procedure, called *laparoscopic lymph node dissection*, which we describe in more detail below. If the lymph nodes are found to be free of cancer, radical perineal prostatectomy is performed shortly thereafter.

Which form of radical prostatectomy is best for you?

That depends on the specifics of your illness and the expertise of your surgeon. Clearly you want your surgeon to perform the type of surgery he or she is most experienced with. You also want a procedure that gives you the best chance of cure with the lowest possible risk. Other factors may also come into play (see Table 8.1). You may feel a risk of having cancer recur is a small

TABLE 8.1: RADICAL PROSTATECTOMY PROCEDURES: PROS AND CONS		
PROCEDURE	**PROS**	**CONS**
Retropubic	• Easy access to lymph nodes for biopsy • If lymph nodes involved, surgery can be stopped • Best for large tumors • Wide surgical margins	• May be hard on men with heart and lung problems
Nerve-sparing	• Least likely to affect potency	• May leave behind some cancerous tissue • Not recommended for larger tumors • Relatively new procedure; long-term benefits not clear
Perineal	• Easiest access to prostate • Shortest operating time, requiring less anesthesia • Safest for men with heart and lung problems • Best for obese men	• No access to lymph nodes • Likely to affect continence and potency • Not recommended for large tumors • Narrow surgical margins

price to pay for maintaining your sexual potency, but another man may not.

QUALIFICATIONS FOR SURGERY

Most surgeons will do a radical prostatectomy on you only if your cancer is stage T1, T2, or T3, confined to the prostate gland and its environs, and if you are in good health and under

---

USUAL QUALIFICATIONS FOR SURGERY

- General good health
- Under 75 years of age
- Stage T1, T2, or T3 tumor (localized)
- Negative bone scan (no metastases)
- Any grade of tumor; high grade (Gleason 8–10) does not rule out surgery so long as cancer is confined to the prostate gland

---

70 or 75 years of age. Your most recent bone scan, if indicated, should show that the cancer has not metastasized. (See box.)

Until recently, experts thought that a man with an aggressive cancer would not benefit from surgery, since a Gleason score of 8 to 10 was assumed to indicate that the cancer had already metastasized. New studies, however, report that even a high-grade cancer may not yet have spread. Consequently, men with aggressive cancer can still hope for a cure, as long as the cancer has not metastasized.

GETTING READY FOR SURGERY

Once you have opted for surgery, you'll naturally be anxious to get it over with. Before proceeding, you should discuss with your doctor the possibility of taking the following steps.

Donating Blood

Improvements in radical prostatectomy techniques have made it a much less bloody operation than in the past. Still, some men will need blood transfusions during the procedure. You could receive blood from another donor, but it is safer to receive your own blood when possible. This is called *autologous blood dona-*

IS SURGERY RIGHT FOR YOU?
(ARE YOU RIGHT FOR SURGERY?)

Before you decide to undergo radical prostatectomy, consider the following questions:

Will surgery cure my cancer?

If your PSA is low and your Gleason score is 6 or less, your cancer may be so slow-growing that it will remain localized and will never become life-threatening. But with a high PSA and a Gleason score of 7 or higher, there is a strong possibility that a localized tumor will spread eventually. Aggressive therapy such as radical prostatectomy offers a good chance of removing the cancer before that can happen.

Am I young enough to benefit from an attempt at a cure?

If, statistically speaking, your chances of living more than ten years are low, then radical prostatectomy may not add significantly to your survival, and there is even a chance that the adverse effects of surgery will affect the quality of your remaining years. But if you are in good health and can expect to live more than ten years, you may be a good candidate.

Am I healthy enough?

Radical prostatectomy is major surgery. It involves anesthesia and puts stress on your body. If you don't suffer from other serious health problems, particularly cardiac or pulmonary diseases, and if you are not especially anxious or fearful about surgery, you may be a good candidate.

Am I willing to live with side effects should they occur?

Your surgeon will do his or her best to ensure that you will not be troubled by incontinence or impotence but cannot guarantee that you won't. If the idea of living with these potential side effects is unbearable, you should consider a nonsurgical treatment.

tion. Your doctor may suggest that you donate blood during the month preceding surgery. Blood keeps for only about forty-five days, so you'll need a firm date for surgery before you begin this process.

Hormone Therapy

Hormone therapy reduces testosterone levels and causes the prostate gland to shrink, which makes the surgeon's job easier. There is also the possibility that hormone therapy can shrink the cancerous tumor itself.

Lymph Node Biopsy

If there's a likelihood that your cancer has spread and you are scheduled to undergo a radical perineal prostatectomy, your doctor may want to perform a lymph node biopsy. The findings of a biopsy will be important for deciding the next step in your treatment.

A lymph node biopsy can be done in one of two ways, depending on the surgeon's preference. The most likely choice will be to make a standard lower abdominal incision and remove pelvic lymph nodes for analysis. Alternatively, your surgeon may decide to perform a *laparoscopic lymph node dissection,* which is a minimally invasive procedure done in the hospital under anesthesia. The surgeon makes several small incisions in your abdomen and inserts a scope to which is attached a video camera. Watching a monitor, the surgeon guides the scope to the lymph nodes and then, using special tools, removes the nodes and sends them to the pathologist. If a biopsy shows that the lymph nodes are positive for cancer, some surgeons will not operate, while others will proceed with surgery followed by radiation or hormonal therapy.

As previously described, if you undergo a radical retropubic prostatectomy, your surgeon can perform a lymph node dissection and biopsy at the beginning of the procedure. This can't be done during a perineal prostatectomy, because this approach does not provide access to the lymph nodes.

RADICAL PROSTATECTOMY, STEP BY STEP

If surgery is your choice of treatment for prostate cancer, ask your doctor to carefully spell out all the possible scenarios beforehand. Make sure, for example, that you understand the circumstances under which the nerve-sparing procedure can and cannot be performed. Establish whether you will undergo an orchiectomy at the time of your prostatectomy. Knowing that your surgeon must make certain decisions based on what he finds at the time of the procedure, and understanding the potential consequences of those decisions, will better prepare you for the outcome.

Days Before Surgery

Before entering the hospital, you'll be asked to stop taking any products that contain aspirin. Aspirin delays the formation of blood clots and can lead to excessive bleeding during surgery. A surprising number of products contain aspirin, including Pepto-Bismol and Alka-Seltzer. Of course, if you're taking aspirin because of blood or heart problems, check with your other doctors first.

If you are banking blood, you will make your last deposit at this time.

Eve of Surgery

During radical prostatectomy there's a risk that an area of the rectum can be inadvertently opened or injured. To prevent infection, you will probably be given a bowel preparation such as an enema. You may be asked to drink a gallon of a saline solution, which induces diarrhea and helps clean out the bowel even further. You will also be given an antibiotic by mouth. You'll take nothing by mouth after midnight on the day before surgery. A clean bowel, combined with the antibiotic, reduces the risk of wound infection.

Day of Surgery

You may be asked to wear special stockings designed to help prevent clots from forming in your veins and escaping to the lungs, where they could cause serious damage or even death. Some hospitals use *pneumatic sequential stockings*, which periodically squeeze your legs to stimulate circulation during and after the surgical procedure.

Anesthesia

Prior to surgery you'll meet your anesthesiologist, who will talk to you about his or her role during the procedure. At this time be sure to mention any problems with or serious reactions to anesthesia that you've had in the past. You may have to undergo blood tests to make sure all is in order for your anesthetic.

You may be given general anesthesia, which will put you completely to sleep; in most cases, when you awaken, you will not remember anything about the surgery.

It is also possible to receive *regional* anesthesia so that you feel nothing from the waist down but remain completely conscious the whole time.

With *spinal anesthesia*, you receive a shot of local anesthetic in the small of your back. The drug penetrates the *dura*, which is the membrane lining the spinal cord, and goes directly into the spinal fluid. Within a few minutes you'll be numb from your waist to your toes. In some cases you will also receive a tranquilizer to help you relax.

With *epidural anesthesia*, the doctor inserts a tiny plastic tube in your back between two vertebrae. The anesthetic travels through this tube and soaks the area outside the dura, producing numbness below where the tube is inserted.

Surgical Prep

Once you are in the operating room your pubic area will be shaved. An intravenous (IV) tube will be inserted into your arm to administer medications and anesthetic; the tube remains in place after the operation so you can receive nutrients and fluids.

The Procedure

RADICAL RETROPUBIC PROSTATECTOMY

The surgeon makes the incision in the lower abdomen and approaches the prostate from behind the pubic bone (*retro* means "behind"). Once inside, the surgeon gently nudges the abdominal organs aside and removes the lymph nodes that are in the most likely path of metastasizing prostate cancer. If the pathologist gives the all-clear sign—no metastases were found in the frozen section—the surgeon proceeds to remove the prostate gland and the seminal vesicles. If there is evidence of cancer in the lymph nodes, most surgeons will stop the procedure. However, some surgeons, believing that the less cancerous tissue left in the body the better, will go ahead with the operation and offer additional (or *adjuvant*) therapy to control the cancer. Once the prostate is out, the surgeon rejoins the urethra to the bladder.

NERVE-SPARING RADICAL PROSTATECTOMY

The surgeon examines the tiny, delicate bundles of nerves and blood vessels that travel along either side of the prostate. If no cancer is found, the surgeon carefully severs the bundles only at those branches where they attach to the prostate. The main connection, between the central nervous system and the penis, stays intact. An operation that spares one bundle is termed *unilateral*; a *bilateral* procedure saves both.

RADICAL PERINEAL PROSTATECTOMY

The surgeon gets to the prostate via the perineum. Lymph node analysis is not done, but the rest of the steps are the same as for the radical retropubic prostatectomy.

Pathology Report

The pathologist studies the prostate shortly after it is removed, cutting the specimen into slices and analyzing them under a microscope. The report indicates whether or not the cancer appears to have been completely removed. A final Gleason score is also assigned. This information helps you and your urologist decide what ongoing treatment you might need.

When prostate cancer is confined to the prostate gland, fewer than one patient in ten experiences recurrence. But if the pathologist finds that disease has spread beyond the prostate, or if the surgical margins are positive (that is, they contain evidence of cancer), then the chance of recurrence is higher. With cure less likely, palliative treatment—hormones, radiation, experimental drugs—may be considered.

Optional Procedures

Your surgeon may have suggested other procedures be done while you're under the knife. Orchiectomy is sometimes performed immediately in patients with lymph node metastases. A hernia can also be repaired.

THE RECOVERY PROCESS

Usually after surgery you will be taken to the recovery room, but if your surgery was complicated or if you are in poor health you may be taken to the intensive care unit, where the medical staff can keep a closer eye on you.

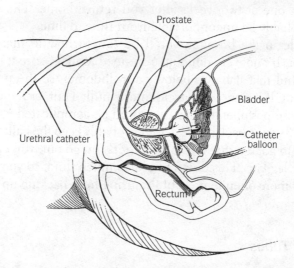

Figure 8.5: Urethral catheter in place, with balloon inflated.

If you've had a general anesthetic, the first step of your recovery is to wake up. As the effects of anesthesia, sedatives, and muscle relaxants wear off, you may feel disoriented. These feelings will pass. Your anesthesiologist will visit you several times to make sure there are no complications.

Your Catheter

When you return to consciousness, you'll no doubt notice that a tube is sticking out of your penis. Meet the catheter, a rubber tube with a balloon attached at one end (Fig. 8.5). The tube goes through the penis via the urethra to the bladder, where the balloon is inflated to keep it in place. The catheter allows urine to drain without burdening your reconstructed urinary tract. The catheter will stay in place throughout your hospital stay and for the first one or two weeks after you return home. The catheter will probably be uncomfortable from time to time.

While in the hospital, you'll be taught how to manage the catheter. It's not very difficult. You need to make sure it is always clean and that it hangs below your abdomen so the urine will drain out. If it were to be accidentally pulled out, or removed too soon, your postoperative course could be complicated.

Once you're back home, you'll probably keep the catheter connected to a large drainage bag. When you go out, you can use a smaller leg bag. This doesn't hold as much fluid, so you need to drain it more often to prevent the urine from backing up into the bladder.

Other Tubes

Drains from the site of the incision are there to remove any fluid that might collect in your wound. You will also still be connected to the IV line until you can keep food and drink down. You'll know that you're on the verge of being discharged when the nurse removes your IV and you begin eating a regular diet.

Pain Management

There are many effective drugs available to take care of any pain you feel after surgery. Recently, thanks to a new pain medication called ketorolac (Toradol), radical prostatectomy patients are going home much more quickly after their operation than they did in the past. Older painkillers often caused severe nausea, making it tough to eat or keep down food and medicine. With ketorolac, many men are able to resume eating much sooner (sometimes even on the day of surgery), which means they can go home sooner.

If you experience pain, or if your pain is not adequately controlled, by all means speak to your caregivers. There is no need for you to suffer unnecessarily. One modern method of dealing with pain is the *patient-controlled pump*. The pump is attached to an IV line and has a button you push to deliver a small dose of narcotic whenever you feel the need. The pump has safeguards to prevent you from using too much medication. This method allows you to get as much pain relief as you need, as soon as you need it. Studies show that patients using the pump often use *less* medication than if they receive injections or pills.

No Heavy Lifting

Until the tissue heals fully, the only thing holding your incision closed is the sutures. To minimize stress on this area, you'll be asked not to lift anything heavier than ten pounds for five or six weeks.

Your First Steps

The day after your surgery, you'll be encouraged to start walking around; at first with the help of a nurse, and later on your own. Exercise is a good way to help prevent blood clots and pneumonia. It also helps keep the digestive system working and eliminates the gas pains many patients consider the most painful aspect of postoperative recovery.

Taking Care of Business

A big milestone on your road to recovery will be your first postsurgical bowel movement. Understandably, considering what they've been through, many men are pretty anxious about this prospect. After surgery, the rectal area can be very sensitive and tender, and many men get dehydrated, which can lead to constipation.

Nonetheless, it's important that you have a bowel movement before going home. You may be given stool softeners and laxatives. Enemas may not be a good idea, because the rectal wall nearest the surgical site can be too weak to withstand the pressure.

POSSIBLE COMPLICATIONS OF
RADICAL PROSTATECTOMY

- Persistent incontinence (3% of total)
- Urethral stricture (5%–10%)
- Damage to ureters (0.1%)
- Impotence (see Table 8.2)
- Cardiovascular problems (1.4%–8%)
- Blood clots in legs; pulmonary embolisms (2.6% or less)
- Rectal injury (less than 0.1%)

Getting Back to Normal

You may be discharged within three to four days after surgery. In most cases, the sooner, the better. Most men find it easier to be more active in familiar surroundings. They sleep better there, too. Once home, you'll be encouraged to take long walks and eat and drink what you like. The sooner you and your body settle back into your routine, the faster you'll recover. For a few months, you may find yourself tiring easily and needing to take naps. Rest is crucial. Surgery has a big impact on your body, and you should give yourself time to recover.

COMPLICATIONS

Like any major surgery, prostatectomy poses a risk of complications and adverse effects (see box). The ones men most fear are incontinence and impotence, which are discussed in more detail in chapters 14 and 15.

Surgical and Anesthetic Risks

The most common surgical problem with radical prostatectomy is blood loss, which is why many surgeons recommend banking your own blood prior to surgery.

TABLE 8.2: IMPOTENCE AFTER RADICAL PROSTATECTOMY (IN MEN POTENT BEFORE SURGERY)		
PROCEDURE	**AGE GROUP**	**RATE OF IMPOTENCE**
Standard radical prostatectomy	All ages	65%–90%
Nerve-sparing, bilateral	Under 60	25%–30%
	60 to 70	40%–50%
	70 and over	70%–80%
Nerve-sparing, unilateral	All ages	59%

Rectal injury occurs in less than 0.1 percent of cases. In these rare instances, a temporary diverting colostomy (allowing waste to exit the body through an opening in the abdominal wall into a bag) can be done to give the rectum time to heal. Later the colostomy will be reversed and normal bowel function restored. Most of the time, however, if a rectal injury occurs, it can be repaired immediately without any delay or change in the postoperative course.

Injury to the ureters (tubes from the kidney to the bladder) is also rare, occurring in about one in a thousand cases.

Urethral Stricture

In 5 to 10 percent of cases, prostate surgery leaves patients with a narrow urethral channel, causing restricted flow of urine. The narrowing, or *stricture*, can be relieved with a procedure called a *dilation*, performed in the physician's office.

Risk of Recurrence and Additional Treatment

In one study, an overall cancer recurrence rate of 12 percent was found after radical prostatectomy. In a Medicare survey of older men, 28 percent had recurrence. Should prostate cancer recur, palliative treatment using radiation or hormone therapy is an option.

Cardiopulmonary Complications

There is a chance that blood clots can form during or after surgery. The incidence of pulmonary embolism or blood clots in the veins is 2.6 percent or less. The risk of these complications increases with age and may be higher in men who have a history of cardiopulmonary problems.

DOES SURGERY WORK?

One way to define success is whether the procedure results in a cure—that is, if the cancer never comes back. A 1992 study found that when the cancer was confined to the prostate, only 2 percent of men had local recurrences within five years after radical retropubic prostatectomy and 1 percent had distant metastases. If the tumor was found in some other part of the tissue specimen (but not beyond that tissue), the rate for local recurrence was 8 percent with 2 percent for distant metastases within five years. If the cancer had spread farther than the surgical margins, the rate of local recurrence was also 8 percent but the rate of metastasis was 30 percent.

Long-term cancer-free survival used to be the only meaningful way to define "cure." The PSA test has changed that. Today, cure can be defined as no detectable PSA level after surgery (PSA <0.1 ng/mL). If your PSA level begins to rise after radical prostatectomy, the procedure may not have resulted in a cure. A small rise may not be clinically significant. Even if it is, there are still many treatment options open to you, as we discuss in chapter 13.

There is no reliable information yet on the success rate of the nerve-sparing radical prostatectomy because the procedure has been available only since the 1980s. Prostate cancer grows so slowly that, as a rule, fifteen years must elapse before we know whether a treatment is effective.

Another measure of success is whether surgery adds years to your life. Here the jury is still out. Some research suggests that men age sixty-five or under who have radical prostatectomy live an average of fourteen months longer than they would have had they chosen watchful waiting.

These statistics apply to large groups of men. You may do considerably better. In any case, fourteen months may not seem like a lot, but if they're *your* months, they can be pretty precious.

VOICES OF EXPERIENCE

"Some men say they opted for radiation because they wanted to avoid the pain of surgery. But the way surgery is done today, I had some discomfort but not a lot of pain. I think where pain is concerned, the biggest factor is mental, not physical. I made my choice because of a double negative. If five years from now I'm sick and facing death, I don't want to look back and regret the fact that I had a chance at a more aggressive treatment but didn't take it."

—Adrian, retired mechanical engineer from Ohio;
had radical prostatectomy at age 60

"I wasn't afraid of dying—I was afraid of *not living.* I didn't want anything to compromise the future I've got carved out for myself. I wanted to do something that would beat the cancer once and for all. After a lot of research and soul-searching, I decided on surgery."

—Virgil, textile sales manager from New Jersey;
had nerve-sparing radical prostatectomy at age 48

"My son's a physician, but he wouldn't give me advice. He told me I had to research it for myself. I finally made the decision to have the surgery because I'm the type who would rather see the prostate in a jar across the room, and know it was out of me for good. My son said, 'Dad, you made the right decision—for *you*.' "

—*Art, retired Air Force officer, Colorado;*
had radical prostatectomy at age 61

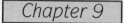

Radiation Therapy

About a hundred years ago, a French scientist carrying a bit of radioactive material in his pocket found that the skin of his hand had become burned. With that accident came the discovery that radiation can destroy human tissue.

Properly harnessed, such destructive power can be directed against cancerous cells. Radiation doesn't kill cancer cells outright. Instead it damages their DNA, hindering their ability to divide and reproduce. As the French scientist found, to his dismay, radiation does the same thing to healthy cells, but those tissues have a greater capacity to recover than do cancer cells.

Like surgery, radiation therapy works best when the cancer is caught at an early stage and is still confined to the prostate gland. As we discuss in this chapter, radiation can be delivered externally, through a device that emits a concentrated beam of energy, or it can be delivered through tiny pellets implanted directly into the prostate. Radiation may be the only treatment you receive, although in some cases it is used in conjunction with hormone therapy or following surgery to destroy any cancer left behind. In advanced cancer, radiation is used to relieve pain.

If you choose radiation therapy, your treatment will be handled by a medical team headed by a radiation therapist, who is an MD or a doctor of osteopathy with specialized training in the administration of radiation therapy. You'll also meet radiation technicians, nurses, and even physicists.

QUALIFICATIONS FOR EXTERNAL-BEAM RADIATION THERAPY

- Life expectancy of 7 to 10 years or more
- Surgery not desired or not possible
- Localized (organ-confined) cancer
- Several weeks' delay after any type of prostatic surgery

EXTERNAL-BEAM RADIATION THERAPY (EBRT)

First introduced in 1956, external radiation has been refined and improved over the years. As the name implies, this approach uses a beam of radiation that originates from outside the body.

You're a good candidate for external radiation if you have a life expectancy of seven to ten years or more, your cancer is localized (confined to the prostate gland), and if you don't want—or can't have—surgery. If your cancer was discovered unexpectedly during another procedure, such as transurethral resection of the prostate, adenomectomy (a procedure for treatment of BPH), or a surgical procedure for relief of bladder outlet obstruction, then you'll have to wait several weeks for the operative site to heal before beginning therapy. This minimizes the risk of incontinence and reduces the scar tissue that can form around the urethra after radiation.

Types of EBRT

Most centers offering EBRT use devices that emit either high-energy X rays or gamma rays, but they produce radiation doses hundreds of times greater than do machines used for diagnostic X rays. One of the major risks associated with this kind of radiation is that some amount of healthy tissue around the prostate inevitably is hit and damaged by the beam. Short-term side effects

---

ALL IN THE NUCLEAR FAMILY

External-beam radiation therapy is made possible by sophisticated machines that produce high-energy subatomic particles. Different machines produce different types of particles, each with its own distinct advantages and disadvantages.

The older cobalt-60 or cobalt-80 machines have inside them a piece of radioactive material that emits particles called neutrons, which the machine gathers and focuses to produce the treatment beam. Old cobalt machines are associated with a higher rate of side effects than the newer linear accelerator machines.

Linear accelerators that generate electron beams are a better source of radiation than cobalt units. These devices don't actually contain any radioactive substances. Instead they produce their own radiation by generating subatomic particles.

---

such as incontinence and long-term side effects such as impotence may result from this damage.

Another, newer approach known as *proton-beam radiation* allows the energy beam to be tightly focused on the prostate and cancer cells where the radiation is most needed. This improved accuracy could mean that when higher doses of radiation are aimed at the tumor, there will be less danger of hitting healthy surrounding tissue, thereby reducing the risk of side effects. Proton-beam radiation requires a detailed, three-dimensional computer image of the target and nearby structures, which is obtained using a CT scan of the area. Sometimes the diameter of the proton beam is too small to encompass the entire prostate, and special filters must be used to adjust the beam. This filtering process decreases some of the benefits of the proton beam.

Proton-beam radiation appears to be a safe and effective form of radiation therapy, but its advantages over conventional radiation are still under investigation. Currently, the treatment is very expensive and available at just a few medical centers.

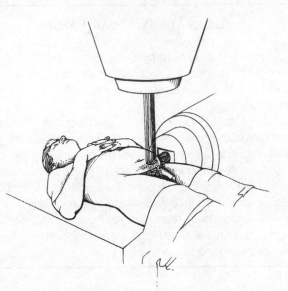

Figure 9.1: Radiation therapy.

Mapping Your Prostate

Think of the radiation beam as a powerful shaft of intense light. Instead of stopping on the surface of your skin, however, this "light" penetrates to tissues located deep inside the body. Your doctors want the light to fall on only the cancerous tissue while keeping the healthy tissue in "shadow."

If your cancer is low grade, radiation will probably be applied to the prostate gland only. But if you have a more aggressive cancer, your doctor may want the beam to treat the entire pelvic region to make sure the radiation also reaches the seminal vesicles and the lymph nodes.

To direct the beam accurately, the care team needs a precise map of your anatomy. You may be asked to undergo CT scans, plain X rays of the pelvis, *urethrograms*, or other tests. Dye is used to make the prostate visible on an imaging machine. The radiology team identifies the target tissue, calculates how much radiation will be needed to eliminate the cancer, and determines which filters will be used.

A man whose cancer is low grade might typically receive a total dose of 6,000 to 7,000 cGy in the course of his treatment. (The cGy—short for centigray—is the standard unit of radiation. One cGy is equal to one rad, which is a more familiar term for radiation dosage.) That works out to about 200 cGy per day, five days a week for six to seven weeks. If the cancer is high grade, the dose might be a total of 5,000 cGy to the pelvic area and 7,000 to the prostate. The dose has to be "diluted"—spread out over time—because it would seriously damage healthy tissue if received all at once.

Before your first dose of radiation, the radiation therapist will draw a target on your body using indelible ink. This target tells the team where to aim the radiation beam. (Be careful that you don't wash this target off, and don't redraw it yourself if it starts to fade. Changing the shape of the target by even a fraction of an inch could cause the beam to hit the wrong place.)

You don't have to be hospitalized to receive EBRT. You simply come into the radiotherapy center at the time of your appointment, lie down on the table, and receive the radiation, which takes only a few seconds (Fig. 9.1). The whole procedure may occupy only ten or twenty minutes of your day.

The duration of your radiation therapy depends on what you and your doctor want to accomplish. If you are attempting to cure or control your cancer, treatment will continue for five to seven weeks. Some therapists give their patients several "rest breaks" of one to two weeks, so the overall delivery time may be closer to ten or twelve weeks overall.

Whatever your weekly schedule, your doctor will always give you the weekend off. This gives the healthy cells a chance to regenerate. Once you've begun your radiation therapy, it's crucial that you let nothing interrupt the schedule your doctors arrange for you. Every treatment session counts.

TABLE 9.1: EFFECTIVENESS OF EXTERNAL-BEAM RADIATION THERAPY	
STAGE AT TREATMENT	**10-YEAR SURVIVAL**
T1 (A)	79%
T2 (B)	66%
T3 (C)	55%
N+, M+ (D)	22%

External-Beam Radiation Therapy: The Pros

EVIDENCE OF EFFECTIVENESS

A study at Stanford University found that eight out of ten men with stage T1 or T2 tumors at the time of radiation treatment were still alive after five years. When the tumor was treated at stage T3, N+, or M+, six out of ten survived five years. A study of nearly 1,000 patients treated with radiation found that nearly 80 percent of men with stage T1 tumors and 66 percent of those with T2 tumors were alive after ten years. Predictably, the rate drops with advanced-stage disease; the rates for stage T3 and stage N+ or M+ cancers were 55 percent and 22 percent, respectively.

Statistics like these indicate that radiation is an alternative to surgery for men with stage T1 or T2 cancer. According to these figures you're just as likely to be alive seven to ten years after treatment whether you've had surgery or external radiation.

Beyond ten years, however, a somewhat different picture emerges, one that many doctors think gives surgery a long-term edge. Some studies, for example, have found that the chance some cancers will grow back after ten years is lower with surgery than with EBRT. However, despite questions about radiation's long-term success, there is widespread agreement that it can effectively control pain and other local symptoms of prostate cancer.

EXTERNAL-BEAM RADIATION THERAPY COMPARED WITH SURGERY FOR PROSTATE CANCER

Pros	Cons
• No surgical risks (hospitalization, bleeding, pain)	• Long, rigid treatment schedule
• Lower risk of impotence	• Separate lymph node dissection procedure necessary if spread is suspected
• Lower risk of incontinence	• Significant fatigue, usually toward end of treatment
• Better for men in poor overall health	• Possible side effects: blood in urine, more frequent bowel movements, diarrhea
• For older men, same life expectancy as with surgery	• Relatively high risk of impotence
• Fewer restrictions on working and being active during course and aftermath of treatment	• Risk of bladder damage: cystitis, scarring, sphincter damage, fistula
	• Risk of rectal damage: irritation, proctitis, bleeding, burning, leakage, fistula
	• Risk of temporary prostate swelling, causing urinary problems that require use of catheter
	• Fear that cancer was left in the body

ADVANTAGES OF RADIATION THERAPY OVER SURGERY

The advantage of external-beam radiation is that it avoids the risks that accompany surgery. There is no anesthesia involved, no transfusions, no cutting, and no significant discomfort. It is a good alternative for someone who does not want surgery, or whose state of health precludes surgery.

Radiation therapy seems to carry a lower risk of impotence than does surgery, but the risk is still significant. There's about a 30 to 40 percent chance that a man who undergoes EBRT will become impotent.

Another plus for radiation is that it is less likely than surgery to cause incontinence. According to some reports, fewer than 5 percent of men receiving radiation will experience incontinence.

Unlike surgery, radiation won't keep you from working or being active during your treatment period. You won't experience any hair loss, except perhaps on your belly where the radiation beam touches your skin.

External-Beam Radiation Therapy: The Cons

One big drawback is the rigid schedule that EBRT imposes. You'll have a treatment session each weekday for six or seven weeks. If you live far from the treatment clinic, this may be difficult to manage. Men who select a treatment center in another part of the country find temporary lodging for the time involved. This can add to the expense of treatment, a cost that is not usually reimbursed by insurance companies.

Another negative is that your lymph nodes do not usually get the same pathologic inspection they do during surgery. If you opt for radiation and there is concern that your cancer has spread, a lymph node biopsy may be recommended as a separate, surgical procedure (see chapter 8 for a description of this procedure).

Toward the end of the treatment period, many patients complain of significant fatigue. Usually this problem subsides over a period of months or years.

As mentioned earlier, the risk of impotence after external-beam radiation is less than after radical prostatectomy, but it is still relatively high—an estimated 30 to 40 percent. If impotence does occur after EBRT, symptoms may occur six months to two years after treatment ends. In contrast, impotence that occurs after radical prostatectomy is apparent very quickly.

Less common side effects are scarring or injury to the muscle fibers at the bladder neck or the external urethral sphincter and bladder problems (cystitis). Symptoms of cystitis may include blood in the urine, a burning sensation when urinating, urgency, or urge incontinence. You can expect the bladder irritation to resolve itself spontaneously over several months. If urinary incontinence becomes a serious and persistent problem, surgical techniques are available to help control it (see chapter 14).

For some men, radiation can cause temporary swelling of the prostate, making urination more difficult. Normally the treatment for such urinary obstruction would be a transurethral resection. But it is not a good idea to have this procedure during EBRT because it increases the risk of side effects such as incontinence. Use of a catheter can overcome urinary blockage, but following radiation, constant use of a catheter increases the chance of scarring. Instead, your doctor may want you to learn how to insert a catheter intermittently, so you can relieve your bladder when needed and keep the catheter out the rest of the time.

A common side effect is *radiation proctitis,* which can be accompanied by pain, bowel frequency, bowel urgency, and occasionally bleeding, chronic burning, or rectal leakage. In most cases these symptoms disappear within three to six months after therapy ends. Occasionally, however, symptoms can become chronic.

In rare cases, a patient will be left with a *fistula,* an abnormal connection between the bladder and the rectum. Fixing a fistula requires surgery, during which a drain is implanted in the bladder through the lower abdominal wall to carry urine to a bag outside the body. Some patients may need a colostomy, a temporary diversion of bowel contents to a collection bag on the abdominal wall.

One drawback to be aware of is that after EBRT, some patients experience a lingering concern that not all the cancer was destroyed. They fear that they have not been cured and that they may be harboring a time bomb. Over the years to come, each ache and pain they experience makes them wonder if the cancer

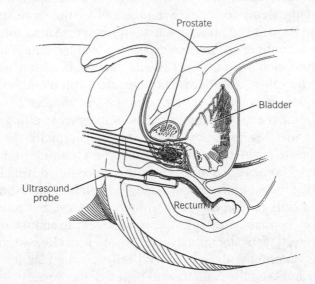

Figure 9.2: Placement of needles during seed implantation.

might have become active and is spreading. While these feelings can affect a man regardless of the type of treatment he chooses for prostate cancer, they are sometimes more pronounced in men who choose radiation.

SEED IMPLANTS

In *seed implant therapy*, tiny radioactive pellets are surgically placed within the prostate gland. Each smaller than a grain of rice, these pellets deliver the dose of radiation right where it is needed, producing only minimal effects on nearby healthy tissue. Doctors sometimes refer to this as *brachytherapy. Brachy* means "short distance," and seed implants do their work within a very confined radius. Another common term is *interstitial* ("in the narrow spaces") *radiation therapy*.

All of the seeds are implanted at the same time. Instead of the short bursts of radiation used in EBRT, seed implants irradiate the cancer continuously, twenty-four hours a day, seven days a week. In most cases, the implants will be left inside the prostate for the rest of the patient's life. However, depending on the radioactive material used, some implants are removed after they have done their job.

To be a candidate for seed implants, your cancer should be stage T1 or T2: localized with no spread of disease to the lymph nodes. Seed implantation is occasionally an option after external radiation fails, but studies are under way to determine whether this might work for some patients. Occasionally EBRT is done in combination with seed implantation, especially if the cancer is close to being stage T3. The best candidate for seed implantation alone has stage T1 or T2a cancer, a PSA level less than 10 ng/mL, and a Gleason score from 2 to 6. Men with smaller prostates who undergo seed implantation have a lower risk of rectal or urinary complications caused by stray radiation. A man with stage T2b cancer, a PSA level greater than 10 ng/mL, and a Gleason score of 7 to 10 is a good candidate for combination therapy.

Materials

Seed implants are made of a number of different radioactive materials, or isotopes. For many years, radioactive gold was literally considered the "gold standard." But this material proved to be especially dangerous to the doctors who handled it. Iodine-125 has been used most frequently over the years, but it is now sharing the stage with the newest entrant, palladium-103.

One measure of a radioactive material's usefulness is its *half-life*, the time it takes for half of the material to "decay," or lose its radiation. The half-life of palladium is seventeen days compared to iodine's half-life of sixty days. But there are other differences between the two, and studies are being conducted to find out which is the better isotope. The more potent the radiation, the greater the possibility of bowel and bladder irritation or long-term injury. Because of this, your radiation therapist will be extremely careful about where the seeds are placed: close enough to the tumor to knock it out, but as far away from healthy neighboring tissues as possible.

Procedure

The implant procedure can be done by your radiation therapist and your urologist working together. You'll be under general or regional anesthesia, so you will need to be hospitalized, though not necessarily overnight.

Modern techniques have made it possible to implant seeds with extreme accuracy (Fig. 9.2). Sometimes an abdominal incision is made between the navel and the pubic bone. More often transrectal ultrasound is used to guide the implant needles as they're inserted through the perineal area between the scrotum and anus. The perineal approach is recommended for permanent implants, while either the abdominal or the perineal route can be used for temporary ones.

In the perineal approach, the physician uses a template, a sheet of metal or plastic with precisely aligned holes, to guide the needles as they're inserted through the area between the scrotum and the anus. No incision is needed. The surgeon watches an ultrasound monitor to help him precisely position each needle deep inside the prostate gland and, if necessary, in the seminal vesicles. Once a needle is in the right location, the seed is injected and the needle withdrawn. The number of seeds ranges from a few dozen to nearly two hundred, with an average ranging somewhere between forty-five and a hundred. The exact number depends on the type of seeds, the size of the prostate, and the extent of the cancer.

During your recovery, you'll feel some discomfort in your bottom. This usually passes in a week or so. You will probably need a catheter for a day to help you urinate. To make sure the cancer has not spread beyond the prostate, you may need to have a separate procedure called a lymph node biopsy (see chapter 8).

In most cases, the seeds will be left in permanently. The seeds stay radioactive for weeks or even months, but the radiation is not a danger to you or to others.

Don't be alarmed if your ejaculate has a dark red or brownish color at first. This is the result of blood in your semen and is to be expected after an implant procedure. It should clear up after several weeks or months and should not be a concern to you or your sexual partner.

Pros and Cons of Seed Implants

PROS

The process of seed implantation takes a lot less time than external-beam radiation therapy. Usually it requires a single procedure lasting one to two hours, compared to weeks of almost daily treat-ments for EBRT. If you live far away from a treatment facility, seed implantation can be a very attractive option. And your odds of remaining potent are better with seed implants than with any other therapy except watchful waiting. The most optimistic reports suggest that if you have not previously had a transurethral resection, the incontinence rate is nearly 0 percent. (But incontinence is frequently seen after a transurethral resection if a patient *previously* had seed implantation.)

Two recent studies indicate that seed implantation is effective treatment for prostate cancer. In a study in Seattle, 97 percent of men treated with seed implants were free of prostate cancer four years after the procedure, as determined by PSA level. A study at Memorial Sloan-Kettering Cancer Center found that 60 percent of men who had undergone seed implants had no evidence of prostate cancer five years after treatment.

CONS

Seed implantation done by this technique is relatively new. The studies cited above are encouraging, but there simply has not been enough time yet to conduct large-scale, long-term comparisons. No study has shown conclusively, for example, that seed

RADIATION PRECAUTIONS

Radiation from your seed implants does not pose a danger to others. The Nuclear Regulatory Commission has determined that if your wife sat in your lap for six weeks, she would receive some kind of measurable dose, but it would still be within the limits of safety.

For the first few months after you've received an implant, some experts suggest that you not have intercourse with any woman who is or might be pregnant. The concern here is that you might expose a fetus to a dose of radiation that could harm its delicate developing tissues.

Also during the first one or two months after seed implantation, you should probably use a condom when you have sex, just in case one of the seed pellets is discharged when you ejaculate. If you do discharge a pellet, don't touch it. Pick it up with a spoon, put it in a glass jar, and return it to your hospital's or clinic's radiation safety control officer.

implantation is *better* than surgery or EBRT. We do know that seed implantation is less likely to be effective for men with large prostates. Even though in some cases seed implantation may not ultimately cure prostate cancer, it can apparently delay its return for years. The choice involves undergoing a therapy with fewer short-term risks and taking a chance that if the cancer returns, it will do so at a point in life where the chances of dying from some other cause are higher.

There is also a wide range of opinion on the risk of side effects from seed implantation. The more pessimistic figures show urinary problems—urgency, frequency, burning, irritation, blood in urine—occurring in one out of four men. Rectal problems—pain, burning, frequency, urgency, and diarrhea—also appear to be a problem in about 5 percent of cases, with higher risk for men whose tumors are more advanced. Interestingly, reported side effects have decreased dramatically in centers where more than five hundred procedures have been performed.

Studies report a rate of impotence between 10 and 30 percent in men who were potent before treatment. To a large extent, the risk depends on the quality of your erections prior to therapy: The better your erections, the more likely you are to retain potency.

Seed implantation treatment also requires that you take certain precautions (see box).

OTHER RADIATION OPTIONS

A combination of external-beam radiation therapy and temporary or permanent seeds can be used to raise the level of radiation to higher levels than either treatment could provide alone. Booster radiation uses seeds implanted either before or after a round of EBRT. It can be an excellent option for men with high-grade cancer, but it is not recommended if the cancer has spread to the lymph nodes. With temporary seeding, the isotope stays in place for a short period of time, during which you will be asked to stay in bed. The seeds are then removed in a second procedure.

Some centers are investigating the use of *hyperthermia therapy*, which applies heat to the tumor, making it even more vulnerable to radiation. If your tumor is stage T2 you may be a candidate for this approach.

Combination therapy uses antiandrogen hormones to shrink the tumor before starting radiation. This may produce better results than radiation alone. Or your doctor may put you on hormones after treatment if radiation alone fails to control your cancer completely.

Sometimes, after a radical prostatectomy, a pathologist will find cancer in the surgical margin of the tissue removed. This could mean that some cancerous tissue was left behind, and that a course of *postsurgical radiation* might be needed to destroy it. If this happens, your radiation team will want to wait a few months for you to recover from the surgery, to give your tissues time to heal.

Remember that a rise in PSA level may indicate the cancer was not eradicated. If radiation is your primary (first-line) therapy, and your PSA rises after treatment, you and your doctor might want to discuss *salvage* procedures that may still be able to eradicate the disease. Sometimes radical prostatectomy is possible after radiation, although many experts don't think this approach does much good. Postradiation surgery seems to work best if both the initial cancer and the recurrence are confined to the prostate gland.

A NEW OPTION: THREE-DIMENSIONAL CONFORMAL THERAPY

An exciting recent innovation, *three-dimensional conformal therapy* delivers higher doses of external radiation in a more carefully controlled fashion. A sophisticated computer measures the volume and area of your prostate in great detail. It then calculates the precise radiation dose needed and creates a three-dimensional computer model of your prostate region. A special body cast is made to hold your body in a precise position so the radiation goes to the same place each time. Then the computer shapes the radiation beam to focus exclusively on the tumor.

Early results are promising. A recent study showed that, compared to conventional radiation treatment, men given conformal therapy were more likely to be alive five years after treatment, to be free of cancer recurrence, to have stable PSA levels, and to have fewer urinary and bowel complications. More studies are needed on larger numbers of men to confirm these results.

Conformal therapy is becoming more widely available in the United States. If you choose this treatment and it is not available close to home, be prepared to travel and spend some time away.

VOICES OF EXPERIENCE

Rick is an active patient, a fifty-two-year-old jazz musician. Not content to rely solely on his doctor's judgment, he studied the different treatments available until he felt confident enough to make his decision.

"I was never of the mind-set that believed 'This cancer has to come out.' I know some people who feel that way. They think if you have it out, you'll be done with it. The fact is, it can come back even after surgery.

"My first urologist mentioned radiation as an alternative to surgery but dismissed it out of hand. That wasn't enough for me. I set about reading and researching and decided my best course would be watchful waiting. When my PSA jumped to 5.2, I knew it was time to do something further. I started on hormone therapy. Meanwhile I discovered a proton beam treatment center nearby. From what I'd learned, I felt this would be a good treatment for me, so that's what I ultimately did. My PSA level has been undetectable for three years. I'm very pleased with my choice, and with my outcome."

"I looked at all the statistics," observed Dick, a computer engineer from Virginia. "I didn't find any that were good enough to convince me to have surgery. The men I met who had seed implants said they felt fine. That was enough to convince me."

Anthony, a sixty-four-year-old retired corporate vice president, participated in a study in which he was given hormone therapy combined with radiation. Three years later his PSA was undetectable. For him, the most reassuring thing about his treatment was the team atmosphere: helpful. "I counsel other men to make sure their doctors talk to each other. All my treatments were done in one facility by doctors who knew each other's methods well. That gave me a feeling of confidence I can't describe to you." He feels that the choice of treatment can't be based exclusively on medical decisions. "You have to be willing to live with the results. If you can't do that with one type of treatment, then choose a different one you can live with. For me, the one-two punch of radiation and hormones was what I needed to feel comfortable."

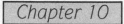

Hormone Therapies

Hormones are chemicals whose job is to keep your body running smoothly. In response to orders from your brain, various organs secrete hormones, which then travel via the bloodstream, sending and receiving messages, switching body functions on or off, speeding things up or slowing them down, and sending back status reports to the brain.

For men with prostate cancer, the most important hormone is one most people know by name: *testosterone.* One of several male sex hormones known collectively as *androgens,* testosterone is the chemical that triggers the masculine body changes of puberty: increased muscle mass, growth of body hair, increase in size of the genitals, deepening of the voice, and so on. It also regulates the level of interest in sex and sexual behavior, moods, and aggressiveness.

Testosterone has another, less welcome property: It stimulates certain kinds of cancer cells, such as those found in many prostate cancer tumors, and causes them to grow. Conversely, if testosterone is removed from the body, any hormone-sensitive tumor usually shrinks. That is why controlling the supply and activity of testosterone is the goal of *hormone therapy*—also known as *androgen-deprivation therapy, androgen blockade* (or *ablation*), and *antiandrogen therapy.*

The quickest, surest way to reduce testosterone is to surgically remove the testicles. The medical term for this procedure is *orchiectomy,* but it is more commonly known as *castration.* By whatever name, men find it an unpleasant prospect. Many won't even consider this option because it threatens their idea of what it means to be a man. Others take a more philosophical view, realizing that the most important virtues of manhood are the products not of hormones but of character.

Traditional means of controlling testosterone levels have been orchiectomy and the use of a synthetic female hormone called diethylstilbestrol (DES). Recently, new drugs have been developed that bring about the same results as orchiectomy while leaving the testicles in place.

HORMONE STRATEGIES

Treatment with hormones is a palliative strategy. While it may *control* the tumor and alleviate symptoms, it will not *cure* prostate cancer, nor is it a substitute for other cure-attempting methods. Your action plan may involve hormone therapy at one or more points.

As a *primary* treatment, hormone therapy may halt the spread of cancer—perhaps not forever, but for a period of time. It may also reduce tumor size, which, in turn, can relieve pain and reduce the need for pain medication. Many men find hormone therapy helps restore appetite and makes them feel stronger and more energetic. The typical candidate for hormone therapy is a man whose cancer has spread to the lymph nodes or to bone. It is often a good choice for an older man for whom radical prostatectomy or radiation therapy is not an option.

Often hormones are used as a *secondary* or *adjuvant* therapy to fight cancer that recurs after treatment.

Some men undergo hormone therapy to shrink the tumor prior to the start of other treatment that is intended to cure the cancer. This approach, known as *neoadjuvant therapy*, may also buy a patient time to consider all his options.

TESTOSTERONE

Testosterone production is a result of a complex chain of events, all regulated by different hormones. Hormone therapies work by

---

INDICATIONS FOR HORMONE THERAPY

Primary therapy:
- Diagnosis of advanced prostate cancer (stage T3 or T4)
- Cancer has spread to lymph nodes and/or bone
- Older patient unable to tolerate other therapy options

Secondary therapy:
- Neoadjuvant: attempt to shrink tumor prior to surgery or radiation is desirable
- Adjuvant: given with or after surgery or radiation

---

interrupting one or more of these events. Becoming familiar with this process will help you understand the options your doctor presents to you.

Your body has two main androgen "factories": the paired testicles and the paired adrenal glands (located just above the kidneys); only a minuscule amount of testosterone comes from other tissues. Each factory is regulated by a slightly different hormone system.

Production by the Testicles

A region in the brain, the hypothalamus, secretes a substance called *luteinizing hormone–releasing hormone* (LHRH). This chemical travels to the neighboring *pituitary gland* and signals it to secrete *luteinizing hormone* (LH). LH then circulates to the testicles, where it signals certain cells (the *Leydig cells*) to release testosterone.

Production by the Adrenal Glands

While about 95 percent of your testosterone is produced by the testicles, most of the rest is the result of androgen production by the adrenals. The process begins in the pituitary gland. While the pituitary is pumping out LH into the bloodstream, it also releases a chemical called *ACTH* (adrenocorticotropic hormone). ACTH circulates to the adrenals, causing them to release androgens. These hormones are converted into testosterone inside cells elsewhere in the body.

What Does Testosterone Do?

When a molecule of testosterone enters the prostate gland, it undergoes a change. An enzyme known as *5-alpha reductase* converts testosterone into an even more powerful version of the hormone called *dihydrotestosterone,* or DHT. Any testosterone left over after this conversion reenters the bloodstream and returns to the hypothalamus. Depending on how much testosterone completes this "feedback loop," the brain will either slow down or speed up the testosterone factory.

Prostate Cancer Cells: A Closer Look

Usually prostate cancer tumors shrink when they are deprived of their testosterone supply. After a while, though, the cancer seems to get used to the absence of hormone. At that point, the tumor can start growing and spreading again.

It is worth taking a moment to understand why.

There are at least three types of prostate cancer cells, each dependent on testosterone to a different degree:

• *Hormone-dependent cells* are extremely sensitive to testosterone; without it they shrink dramatically and quickly.

• *Partially dependent cells* are less reliant on hormone; without it they may shrink, but not as much or as fast as their hormone-dependent brothers.

• *Hormone-independent cells* are completely unaffected by the presence or absence of testosterone.

No two men with prostate cancer have exactly the same proportion of these types of cells in their tumors.

Over time, the proportion of different cell types can change, and this proportion determines the tumor's response to hormone treatment. If all cancer cells were hormone-sensitive, then hormone therapy could stop tumor spread permanently and could result in a cure. Unfortunately that's not the case. It's those hormone-*independent* cells that make prostate cancer so difficult to control. They continue to multiply until they become the largest segment of the cancer cell population. Once they dominate the scene, the cancer becomes insensitive—or *refractory*—to hormone therapy.

TREATMENT STRATEGIES

The use of just one method of hormone manipulation is called single-agent therapy, or *monotherapy*. When two or more methods are involved, it's known as *combination hormone therapy*. The pros and cons of the individual strategies are summarized in Table 10.1. Let's discuss the single-agent methods first.

Single-Agent Therapies

ORCHIECTOMY
Surgical castration is a straightforward procedure that can be done under general, spinal, or even local anesthetic. Sometimes it is performed in combination with radical prostatectomy. The doctor makes a small incision in the front of the scrotum, brings the testicles out through the opening, and severs the testicular cord to which they are connected.

Pros of Orchiectomy: Orchiectomy gets quick results: Within hours, testosterone levels fall by as much as 95 percent. Most men undergoing only orchiectomy go home the day of their surgery. It is the most convenient of all the hormonal therapies: no monthly

| TABLE 10.1: HORMONE THERAPIES: PROS AND CONS |||
TREATMENT	PROS	CONS
Orchiectomy	• Quick and effective • No ongoing drug treatment • Relatively inexpensive	• Does not eliminate adrenal androgens • Psychological impact • Impotence • Loss of libido • Hot flashes
Estrogen (DES)	• Effective • Avoids surgery	• Loss of libido • Risk of heart attack, stroke, blood clots • Breast enlargement • Breast tenderness
LHRH agonists (leuprolide, goserelin)	• As effective as orchiectomy, without surgery • Low risk of cardiovascular side effects • Low risk of breast enlargement	• Risk of tumor flare • Impotence • Loss of libido • Hot flashes • Does not eliminate adrenal androgens • Psychological impact
Antiandrogens (flutamide, bicalutamide)	• Avoids surgery • Blocks adrenal androgens • Reduces risk of testosterone flare caused by LHRH agonist • Most effective used in combination with surgical or medical castration	• Occasional breast enlargement, breast tenderness • Diarrhea • Liver toxicity

injections, no pills. Often it is the cheapest method, requiring a one-time surgical fee instead of ongoing monthly bills for physician-supervised injections or expensive oral medications.

Surgical castration can be an especially good choice for men who need rapid relief from severe symptoms of advanced cancer. Because hormone levels fall so quickly, it is often the best treatment for men with metastases in the spinal column who are at serious risk of paralysis.

Cons of Orchiectomy: The most serious adverse effect of castration and other hormonal therapies is the impact on sexuality. Following orchiectomy, close to 90 percent of men experience impotence and loss of sexual desire.

Up to 40 percent will experience hot flashes—moments of intense body heat resulting in severe discomfort and sweating. These are the same types of hormonal events that women experience at menopause or following removal of the ovaries. Some patients will find relief by taking megestrol acetate (Megace) or clonidine (Catapres), a medication usually used for treatment of high blood pressure.

Nor does orchiectomy eliminate male hormones completely; remember, some are still produced by the adrenal glands. If your cancer is fast-growing and contains chiefly hormone-insensitive cells, you may need additional treatments. Overall, hormonal therapies (including orchiectomy) fail to work in perhaps one case out of five. To find out if their prostate cancer is hormone-sensitive before attempting orchiectomy, some men are put on a drug regimen that medically reduces testosterone levels. If this approach controls the cancer, it's a good indication that orchiectomy may also work.

LHRH AGONISTS

These agents accomplish the same goal as castration—eliminating the testicular source of testosterone—but they work chemically, rather than surgically. They are classified as *analogs*, meaning they are man-made chemicals. An *agonist* is a chemical that produces the same effects as natural substances. Thus an *LHRH-agonist analog* is a synthetic chemical that has effects similar to natural LHRH.

The process by which LHRH agonists work is complex. Normally, the body's own LHRH sends signals to the pituitary in *pulses*, somewhat like the "ping" of sonar. When the pituitary receives the signal, it releases an amount of LH, which then triggers testosterone production in the testicles. In contrast, an LHRH agonist sends a *constant* signal to the pituitary—more like a steady hum than an intermittent ping. At first the pituitary reacts by sending out constant high levels of LH, which in turn leads to increased testosterone production. Over the course of a few weeks, the body's testosterone that returns to the hypothalamus indicates that the testosterone supply is high and the body shuts down the factory. Even in the absence of testosterone production, the LHRH agonist continues to "jam" the signal to the pituitary. The result: Once testosterone production stops, the LHRH agonist keeps it from starting up again.

The two main LHRH analogs are leuprolide (Lupron) and goserelin (Zoladex). They are administered by injection either once a month or by a longer-acting three-month injection.

Pros of LHRH Agonists: LHRH agonists are extremely effective, bringing testosterone levels down to the same range achieved by castration. Compared to such other hormone therapies as DES, LHRH agonists pose a lower risk of cardiovascular side effects, breast enlargement, and nipple sensitivity.

Cons of LHRH Agonists: Lack of testosterone, whether the result of surgical or medical (drug-induced) castration, can cause impotence. Hot flashes are a common side effect. Also, as noted, use of LHRH agonists causes a burst of testosterone that lasts about three weeks following the start of therapy. Because prostate cancer cells are so responsive to testosterone, this three-week burst can stimulate tumor growth. *Tumor flare*, as this phenomenon is called, is very dangerous if the cancer is advanced, especially if it has metastasized to the spine. In rare cases, the tumor growth caused by a flare could damage the spinal cord and lead to paralysis. Some doctors will give patients oral antiandrogens to block the rise in testosterone during this time.

ESTROGEN (DES)

DES (diethylstilbestrol) is an analog, or synthetic form, of estrogen, the main female hormone. Treatment with DES blocks testosterone production by preventing the release of LHRH from the hypothalamus. Testosterone levels usually fall to low levels within fourteen days. DES often causes breast enlargement and breast tenderness. The doses used in clinical practice carry some risk of such cardiovascular side effects as heart disease, fluid retention, and blood clots. For many years, DES was the only hormonal alternative to orchiectomy. It is used less commonly now that other drugs are available.

Combination Hormone Therapy

No single-agent hormone therapy can completely stop androgen production. By bringing several different therapies to bear on the problem, however, you break the androgen cycle at multiple points. That's the goal of combination hormone therapy: *total androgen blockade*. The one-two punch: First eliminate testosterone, using either surgical castration or LHRH agonists. Then use an antiandrogen to block any adrenal male hormones from reaching cancerous cells.

Antiandrogens are drugs that block male hormones (androgens) from reaching and acting on prostate cancer cells. Instead of causing testosterone levels to fall, antiandrogens actually allow them to rise. But that doesn't matter, for two reasons. First, antiandrogens work by creating a barrier around hormone-dependent cells. Unable to absorb the testosterone they need, those cells can't use testosterone to grow. Second, antiandrogens are used in combination with orchiectomy or LHRH agonists to reduce the supply of male hormones.

HORMONE THERAPIES

To lower testosterone levels:
- Surgical castration—orchiectomy
- Medical castration (drug therapy)
  - Estrogens (DES)
  - LHRH agonists (leuprolide, goserelin)

To block androgens from prostate cancer cells:
- Antiandrogens
  - Flutamide (Eulexin)
  - Bicalutamide (Casodex)
  - Cyproterone acetate (Cypteron, Androcur)

Combination hormone therapy (total androgen blockade):
- Orchiectomy or LHRH agonist, plus antiandrogen
  (e.g., flutamide, bicalutamide)

The most widely used antiandrogens in the United States are flutamide (Eulexin) and bicalutamide (Casodex).

Ketoconazole (Nizoral), a drug used to fight fungal infections, has some antiandrogen effects. Though not approved for treating prostate cancer, some physicians find it useful when other therapies have failed.

There is also a family of *steroid antiandrogens* that work by preventing testosterone from reaching prostate cells. One agent, megestrol acetate (Megace), is sometimes given to men who don't respond to LHRH agonists. Medroxyprogesterone (Depo-Provera) is another member of this family. And a drug not available in the United States, called cyproterone acetate (Cypteron; Androcur), is being used either alone or as part of a combination regimen for the palliative treatment of high-stage cancer.

One of the most important measures of successful cancer treatment is whether it increases life expectancy. The facts aren't all in yet, but it appears that combination hormone therapy can extend survival by seven to twelve months or more, compared to other treatments.

Like all medical therapies, combination hormone therapy has its drawbacks. It is expensive, and it can occasionally cause breast enlargement and tenderness, diarrhea, and, in some men, liver damage. These problems can be serious enough to require stopping treatment. The steroidal antiandrogens can cause weight gain, blood clots, and nausea; in general, they tend to lose their effectiveness when used on a long-term basis.

Dosing Strategies

Neoadjuvant therapy uses hormones as a prelude to surgery or radiation. If primary treatment has to be delayed for some reason—the onset of another illness, for example—neoadjuvant treatment can temporarily control the tumor's growth. More often, though, its goal is to make the primary therapy more effective by shrinking the tumor beforehand. One study showed that three to six months of neoadjuvant therapy is necessary to produce the maximum reduction in PSA levels. There is also some evidence that this strategy may make it easier during radical prostatectomy for surgeons to achieve negative margins—that is, to remove tissue that on pathologic exam shows no sign of cancer at the edges.

Adjuvant therapy refers to hormonal treatments given during primary therapy or after treatment is completed.

Scientists are conducting studies to see if the following dosing option might be effective: When the desired low levels of PSA are achieved, hormone therapy is stopped; if levels rise, treatment starts again. This strategy, called *intermittent dosing*, might offer several advantages: The quality of life improves when a man can look forward to having periods of renewed sexual function. What's more, the cost of treatment is lower.

An even greater advantage may be increased survival. Laboratory evidence suggests that hormone-insensitive prostate cancer cells develop only *after* the supply of testosterone is cut off. If so, then periodically restoring testosterone production through intermittent dosing may reduce the opportunity for these cells to proliferate. This means that hormone therapy might be more effective for longer periods.

Other scientists argue, however, that there is no advantage to intermittent therapy and that it may even be counterproductive. They believe that stopping treatment only gives the cancer time to grow and metastasize, and so they feel the best approach is to keep therapy going continuously until it is no longer effective. Hopefully, studies now under way will help resolve the debate.

EFFECTIVENESS OF HORMONE THERAPY

Combination therapy seems to work better than any single-agent strategy. Exactly how *much* better is still an open question. Overall, between 40 and 60 percent of men treated with hormones experience some improvement of their clinical symptoms. Up to 80 percent report relief of pain and discomfort. More than 25 percent of men with metastatic high-stage prostate cancer who receive hormone therapy as their definitive therapy are still alive after five years.

The other side of those figures is that almost 75 percent are not alive after five years. This underscores the point that advanced prostate cancer is a serious and lethal disease. Hormone therapy is a tool, and often a very effective one, for improving the quality of life for many men, and extending life for some. It is not, however, a cure.

Hormone therapy remains a viable option when your primary treatment has reached the limit of what it can do for you. If your PSA rises after radiation or surgery, or if you start to experience pain from metastatic cancer, hormone therapy will often help. For advanced prostate cancer, nothing works as well as hormone therapy.

VOICES OF EXPERIENCE

Making the choice to have an orchiectomy was a tough one for Jim, a former electrical engineer now living in Washington. "I can talk about it now, even joke about it," he says. "I sometimes say that I'm a steer instead of a bull. But I couldn't talk about it at first. I was as bad as the rest of us men. My attitude was, 'Just clam up. Don't tell anybody anything. It's too embarrassing.' Well, now I say the hell with it. I tell everyone, because I figure I can help somebody get diagnosed earlier."

Don, a former businessman, was so impressed by the level of medical care he received during his treatment for prostate cancer that he decided to switch careers. Recently, at age forty-nine, he graduated from nursing school. Five years ago he had neoadjuvant therapy to shrink his tumor before undergoing radical prostatectomy. "The first six months of hormonal therapy I had no libido. But the treatment had one unexpected benefit: It improved my driving. No kidding! It made me less aggressive, which is one of the accidental blessings of the whole thing. I don't know if it was the hormonal therapy, or just facing my mortality, but I found myself less judgmental than I used to be. My wife and I became better friends than we were before, because we had to discover other things to do together besides have sex. If it weren't for the cancer itself, I'd say it this was a good experience—a good period of my life."

Fred, a former assembly worker in a farming-equipment factory, chose an orchiectomy at age seventy partly because he wanted what he calls "a permanent partial cure," and partly because he felt the combination hormone therapy was prohibitively expensive. "I'm retired and living on social security. I didn't think we could afford it very easily. My doctor said the effect of my orchiectomy was my voice wouldn't change and I'd still have to shave. And he was right, of course. As far as the sexual aspects, on me it's easy, because I have no sexual drive now. But it's harder for my wife because she still has those feelings. I feel like I'm less aggressive and I have more patience than I used to. My wife says she notices it too."

Chapter 11

Cryosurgery

We protect our bodies against frostbite because we know excessive cold can kill tissue. Cryosurgery puts the destructive quality of cold to medical use. First developed in the early 1960s, the procedure—also known as *cryoablation* or *cryotherapy*—uses probes to flash-freeze diseased tissue. Initially, hopes were high that the technique might be valuable in treating cancers located within organs such as the prostate. But cryosurgery did not always destroy tumors fully, and often they grew back. Such side effects as incontinence and fistulas (unwanted passages or links between the urethra and rectum) were also frequent. Meanwhile, improvements in surgery and radiation therapy for prostate cancer caused cryosurgery to fall from favor.

In the last few years, improvements in technology have renewed interest in the technique. When it was first developed, cryosurgery was a "blind" procedure. Now, cryosurgeons can actually see what they are doing, thanks to the images provided by transrectal ultrasound. New surgical tools and techniques reduce the risk of excessive tissue damage. Such refinements improve the accuracy with which cryosurgeons can freeze the targeted tissue while avoiding injury to the surrounding normal tissues.

Despite these advances, modern cryosurgery is still in its infancy. Studies are under way to determine its effectiveness in the treatment of prostate cancer. For the most part, cryosurgery is still an experimental approach. It holds promise, because men may tolerate cryosurgery more easily than other invasive procedures, and the technique may have a lower incidence of certain side effects than some other treatments. On the other hand, researchers worry that the procedure may not kill all the cancerous cells, thus increasing the risk of recurrence when compared to other treatments.

ARE YOU A CANDIDATE?

If cryosurgery is to have any chance of curing prostate cancer—which is by no means certain yet—it must be done while the tumor is still confined to the prostate, before it has spread. If you have already had a transurethral resection, cryosurgery can still be an option, but your now-smaller prostate will make the procedure more difficult to perform with accuracy. You can also consider cryosurgery if you've already had radiation therapy or if you have other medical conditions that make it difficult for you to tolerate surgery or radiation. Cryosurgery is not recommended for a man with an enlarged prostate, because the risk is higher that some of the tissue may not become adequately frozen.

PROCEDURE

When first developed, cryosurgery was an "open" procedure. This means the operation required an incision large enough to expose the prostate to the surgeon's view, allowing reasonably accurate placement of the cryoprobe. However, the surgeon could only make an educated guess as to whether the desired result was being accomplished. Often the probe was not placed properly or did not get cold enough to destroy the tissue. Results were disappointing.

Things have improved considerably. If you elect to have cryosurgery, you will be given regional or general anesthesia. To guard against accidentally freezing the urethra, a heated catheter is inserted to insulate the urethra from cryosurgery's freezing cold. Tiny incisions are made between the scrotum and the anus. Using transrectal ultrasound images of the prostate's interior as a

QUALIFICATIONS FOR CRYOSURGERY

- You have localized prostate cancer.
- You have already had unsuccessful radiation therapy.
- You have medical conditions that preclude other treatments.
- Your prostate is relatively small.

guide, the surgeon inserts three to five hollow tubes inside the gland and the seminal vesicles. The surgeon then slides the probes through the tubes until they reach their predetermined locations, making sure to place the probes so as to avoid damaging the rectum, bladder, or urinary sphincter (Fig. 11.1).

The cryoprobe itself is a thin tube that is completely insulated except for four centimeters at the tip. When liquid nitrogen is pumped through the cryoprobe, the tip gets extremely cold. The liquid nitrogen never touches any part of your body; it is used only to lower the probe tip to the correct temperature (−192° C).

The cryoprobe creates a small "ice ball" of frozen prostate tissue around its tip. During the procedure, the urologist (or a radiologist) watches the ultrasound monitor as the ice ball grows. When the ball reaches the desired size, the physician shuts off the freezing action and retracts the probe. The ultrasound monitor helps the medical team see that all the tissue targeted for destruction has been destroyed, and that no damage occurs to the surrounding area.

Modern techniques allow precise placement of the cryoprobes and sophisticated temperature control. Compared to cryosurgery's pioneering days, the risk of damage to the bladder and the rectum is lower.

Evidence suggests that cryosurgery may work better on small tumors. Before the procedure, your doctor may want you to un-

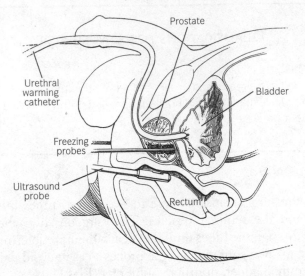

Figure 11.1: Cryosurgery for prostate cancer.

dergo a course of hormone therapy to shrink your tumor. A typical regimen lasts three to six months and involves monthly injections and daily pills. The effects of hormone therapy are temporary. As soon as you discontinue treatment, your hormone levels will return to normal and most or all side effects, such as hot flashes and loss of sex drive, will disappear. (For more information about hormone therapy, see chapter 10).

STEPS IN THE PROCESS

Treatment centers handle cryosurgery in slightly different ways. In a typical scenario, several weeks before your procedure, your doctor will ask you to undergo a bone scan to make sure your cancer has not spread. If it has, cryosurgery will probably not help you and you'll need to consider other treatments. During a preadmission workup, you'll receive a chest X ray, an electrocardiogram, and blood tests.

Although cryosurgery requires a stay in the hospital, you may not have to be admitted until the day of the procedure. The night before you check into the hospital, you should abstain from food and drink after midnight. In the morning you'll be asked to give yourself a saline enema (or two) until you achieve what is euphemistically called "clear results." Before the procedure, you'll be given a sedative and perhaps other medications. You'll then receive a spinal or general anesthetic.

An intravenous tube is inserted so you can receive fluids or medications. A catheter will also be placed in the bladder. This device, known as a *suprapubic catheter,* will remain in place for several weeks after the procedure to help with your recovery. The entire procedure takes only about an hour or two. A few stitches will close up the incisions.

During recovery, while the anesthetic is wearing off, you'll be given pain medications if necessary. You will be encouraged to get out of bed and stand for a few minutes. Some treatment centers will have you wear special support stockings for a day. These apply pressure to your legs to stimulate circulation and prevent blood clots from forming. Your IV tube will remain in place for a while to prevent dehydration. Once your caregivers are sure you can keep liquids down, they'll remove it.

The day after the procedure, you'll be allowed to remove the support stockings. You will also be encouraged to start moving around more in your room and in the hallways.

You are likely to have significant swelling and bruising of your scrotum following the procedure. The swelling will probably disappear within a week or two. To ease the discomfort and the swelling, you can lie flat on your back with a towel under your scrotum. The use of an athletic supporter or ice packs may also help.

Your caregivers will give you explicit instructions on what to do when you get home. It is essential that you understand how to maintain your suprapubic catheter before you are discharged.

A conventional catheter is a tube that is inserted through your penis into your bladder and which drains urine continuously into a plastic bag. The suprapubic catheter you wear after cryosurgery is very different. Instead of being inserted through your penis, the drain tube goes into the bladder through the wall of your abdomen. The device is necessary because after cryosurgery the prostate can swell, making voiding difficult. With the suprapubic catheter in place, urine can escape when necessary.

Because of its placement, the suprapubic catheter may irritate the bladder wall and cause it to contract, giving you the sensation of needing to urinate. Although the contractions may be uncomfortable, they are normal and not serious so long as the urine continues to drain. If the contractions persist, you should notify your doctor, who can prescribe medication to relax your bladder.

It is important to resume urinating normally as soon as your doctor recommends it. Whenever possible, close off the catheter by clamping it and attempt to urinate normally. If you can't void comfortably or in the usual way, you can simply reattach the bag and let the urine drain into it. The goal, though, is to spend as much time as possible off the catheter, hopefully a little longer each day. When your urination returns to normal (typically after a week or two), the doctor simply removes the catheter tube. The hole in the bladder closes by itself; no special procedure is needed.

PROS AND CONS OF CRYOSURGERY

At this time, the benefits and disadvantages of cryosurgery are hard to assess. Researchers don't have enough long-term experience with the procedure to judge its effectiveness accurately. Whether cryosurgery actually cures prostate cancer, or whether it is better for relieving symptoms, is still an open question. Until more studies are done, more men have had the proce-

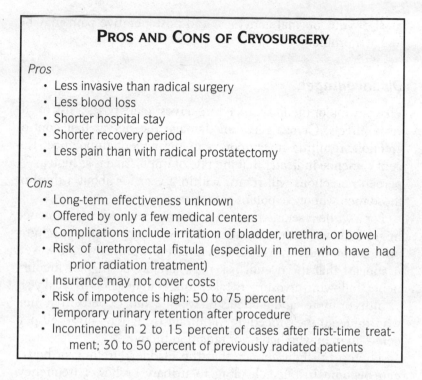

PROS AND CONS OF CRYOSURGERY

Pros

- Less invasive than radical surgery
- Less blood loss
- Shorter hospital stay
- Shorter recovery period
- Less pain than with radical prostatectomy

Cons

- Long-term effectiveness unknown
- Offered by only a few medical centers
- Complications include irritation of bladder, urethra, or bowel
- Risk of urethrorectal fistula (especially in men who have had prior radiation treatment)
- Insurance may not cover costs
- Risk of impotence is high: 50 to 75 percent
- Temporary urinary retention after procedure
- Incontinence in 2 to 15 percent of cases after first-time treatment; 30 to 50 percent of previously radiated patients

dure, and more time has passed, we won't be able to give you the answers you deserve. Meanwhile, here's a summary of what is known.

Benefits

One clear advantage is that cryosurgery is less invasive than radical prostatectomy. The incisions are smaller, posing less risk of damage to other tissues and a lower risk of blood loss during the operation. After radical prostatectomy, you may have to stay in the hospital for three to seven days, but after cryosurgery you might go home after only one or two days. Your general recovery is faster, too. Within a week you can resume most of your normal activities, and postoperative pain may be less of a problem.

Disadvantages

Like any major medical procedure, cryosurgery poses a risk of adverse effects. Cryosurgery can damage the nerves that control erection, resulting in temporary or permanent impotence. Recent evidence indicates that the rate of impotence is as high as 75 percent; erections will return within a year for about a third of those men who were potent before cryosurgery.

For a while it seemed as if the risk of permanent incontinence might be lower with cryosurgery than with radical prostatectomy or radiation therapy. As more men have the procedure, however, it appears that the overall risk may actually be higher. Incontinence following cryosurgery takes longer to develop (typically six months or more) and it affects between 2 and 15 percent of men who undergo the procedure. The rate is higher—up to 50 percent—in men who had prior radiation therapy.

There is a slight chance that the bladder, urethra, or bowel can become irritated, leading to urinary or bowel frequency, blood in urine or stools, or burning and pain when urinating. A few men will be troubled by a serious problem called *urethrorectal fistula,* which means an abnormal passage between the prostatic urethra and the rectum. In one study this occurred in 2.4 percent of cases, but most of those affected were men who had prior radiation treatment, which may have weakened the tissue. Fistulas can be a very difficult problem to correct, but the damage can be repaired through surgery.

In addition, about 50 percent of cryosurgery patients experience swelling of the penis or scrotum that may last a week or two. About as many will also experience numbness in the tip of the penis, which can persist for up to six months.

One other problem: Because cryosurgery is still considered experimental, many insurance companies refuse to pay for it.

EFFECTIVENESS OF CRYOSURGERY

Cryosurgery has one big disadvantage that must be taken into consideration: We don't know if it works. If it does work, we don't know how well. Some evidence seems to suggest that its long-term efficacy may compare favorably to standard treatments. But there's still a lot we don't know. Modern cryosurgical techniques have only been around since the early 1990s; as of this writing, we don't even have five-year survival statistics available.

There is unsettling evidence suggesting that some prostate cells—healthy ones as well as cancerous ones—may survive the procedure. If true, this poses a serious risk that the cancer will recur. In two-year follow-up studies, 20 percent of cryosurgery patients had a positive biopsy and about half had elevated PSA levels, indicating that cancer was left behind.

While some practitioners and patients view cryosurgery as a reasonable alternative, it must still be considered experimental.

VOICES OF EXPERIENCE

"It seemed like everyone I talked to wanted to push a radical prostatectomy on me. And they told me I'd be impotent for sure," complained George, a sixty-three-year-old factory supervisor from Los Angeles. "I liked the idea of cryosurgery because it was the least invasive. So I went to several urologists to find out more." But he was surprised—and frustrated—to find out how little is known of this relatively new procedure. "Very few of these doctors knew anything about cryosurgery. I had trouble even finding a hospital that would do it. I checked out an online prostate users' group and found a list of hospitals doing the procedure. Turned out there was one near me."

After all that, George still had one more hurdle to clear. "I had to contend with my health insurance company. Nobody there had ever heard of cryosurgery, and they wouldn't pay. So my wife went to bat for me. She appealed the decisions when they turned us down. Eventually she arm-twisted them into paying for the treatment. I guess we wrote better letters than they did."

Cryosurgery was also the first choice for Tony, a sixty-six-year-old automotive designer from Michigan. But his insurer also refused to cover the treatment. He planned to mortgage his house to pay the costs, but changed his mind when he realized that an unexpected complication could wipe him out financially. "Right now my only options are a radical prostatectomy—which my doctor says is not a good idea for me because of my other health problems—or radiation, which is a big problem because the nearest radiation center is a hundred miles away."

Chapter 12

Alternative Approaches to Treatment

In this chapter we'll briefly discuss therapies (other than surgery, radiation, and hormones) that have been used at one time or another in the fight against prostate cancer. Topics here cover a broad spectrum of healing philosophies and approaches. What they all have in common, however, is that *they have not yet been shown conclusively to be of great value in the treatment of prostate cancer.*

Your doctor may offer you some of the chemotherapy drugs here. All of these approaches have been evaluated for safety; many of the drugs we mention are used effectively to treat other forms of cancer or other medical problems. These methods, however, have not yet been shown to be effective in the treatment of prostate cancer, or their effectiveness is less than that of other, established therapies. This does not mean they are useless. While they may not arrest or cure prostate cancer, they may offer some degree of relief from symptoms.

Our purpose in this chapter is to make you aware of *all* the options out there, but with some important caveats:

• Just because a choice is available does *not* mean the choice is a good one.

• The glowing testimony of a few people is *not* proof that a treatment works.

• When dealing with life-and-death issues such as prostate cancer, enthusiasm is no substitute for science.

CHEMOTHERAPY

Chemotherapy is the use of drugs to fight cancer. There are no known drug treatments that can *cure* prostate cancer at any stage. Some drugs have been approved for palliative use in men with high-stage cancer. These drugs sometimes slow the growth of the tumor or prevent cells from metastasizing. In most cases, drugs are an option after hormone therapy has been tried and found either to have no effect or to be no longer effective.

Chemotherapy is commonly used in many other cancers; prostate cancer is an exception. If your doctors don't offer you drugs, or if they don't spend much time talking with you about these options, it's not because they're hiding anything from you. It's because there just aren't any proven options available at this time. Many drugs that have even a glimmer of promise are still experimental and not approved for general use. Some aren't even available in this country. The situation may change in the future, as we come to know more about the nature of prostate cancer and discover new drugs or find effective ways to use old ones. In the meantime, here's a quick rundown on some of the main ways drugs can affect prostate cancer.

Altering the Cancer Cell's Life Cycle

Some drugs interfere with the various biologic processes the cancerous cell must carry out to live.

GROWTH

Suramin works by blocking *growth factors*, which are proteins that stimulate tumor cell division. Originally developed as a treatment for parasite infections, suramin may also work by inhibiting the effect of male hormones on prostate cancer cells. Some studies found that up to 30 percent of men taking suramin experience relief of bone pain, accompanied by lower PSA levels (falling as much as 75 percent over eight weeks). Such response may last only three months or so. The drug is given as a weekly injection or as a continuous IV infusion. Possible side effects include damage to the nerves or kidneys and lowered immunity against other diseases.

HORMONAL ACTIVITY

Drugs such as octreotide acetate (Sandostatin) are prescribed for people who have excess amounts of the body's natural growth hormone. Research is under way to determine whether these drugs might also inhibit the growth factors that promote prostate cancer tumors. Studies are also looking at whether high doses of lovastatin, a drug widely used for treatment of high serum cholesterol levels, achieve this effect.

AGGRESSIVENESS

As you know, your Gleason score describes how aggressive your tumor is. Cells from aggressive tumors are less differentiated, meaning that the tumor looks less and less like the prostate tissue it came from. If we can somehow alter the differentiation process, we might keep prostate cancer from becoming aggressive. Drugs under study for this purpose are phenylacetate given as an IV infusion and compounds derived from retinoids (essentially vitamin A)

BLOOD VESSEL DEVELOPMENT

Scientists are also studying drugs that interfere with the tumor's ability to generate its network of blood vessels. By starving the tumor of its blood supply, we may be able to keep it from progressing.

ENZYME ACTION

Finasteride (Proscar) is used in the treatment of benign prostatic hyperplasia. It works by inhibiting the prostate cell enzyme called 5-alpha reductase. This enzyme converts molecules of testosterone into their active form, DHT. Researchers are studying Proscar to learn whether it might keep prostate cancer from developing in men who are at risk (see page 43).

Killing Cancer Cells

Estramustine, sold under the brand name Emcyt, is a combination of estradiol and nitrogen mustard. At the time of this writing, it is the only drug approved specifically for palliation of progressive or metastatic prostate cancer. The presence of estradiol, a form of estrogen, helps block the response of tumor cells to male hormones. Estramustine is often combined with another drug, such as vinblastine or etoposide, to shrink tumors. The most common side effects of estramustine are breast tenderness and breast enlargement, which affect more than 60 percent of the men who take the drug.

Methotrexate is a cytotoxic (cell-killing) drug used to treat many types of cancer. Some evidence suggests that it may work against prostate cancer if injected into or near the organ.

Other drugs under study include cyclophosphamide, methylglyoxal, and a combination regimen of novantrone or adriamycin plus 5-fluorouracil (5-FU).

Relieving Symptoms

Pain is probably the biggest concern of men whose prostate cancer is high stage. Among the most promising treatments for pain are *radioisotopes*, compounds that emit low, safe levels of radiation. The best known of these is strontium-89, sold as Metastron. Other examples include rhenium-186 and samarium-153. Some treatment centers are experimenting with combinations of a radioisotope and cis-platinum, a chemotherapy drug. Another approach combines samarium-153, which appears to have some cell-killing ability, with aminophosphoric acid, which acts by attaching itself to cancer cells. The combination of these two drugs is lethal to the cell.

Corticosteroids—hormones produced by the adrenal glands—can control cancer-associated pain in some men. Unfortunately, synthetic corticosteroid use also carries the risk of a host of un-

---

DEALING WITH PAIN

For most people with advanced prostate cancer, pain relief is probably the top priority. If you experience pain, be sure to tell your doctor. Some men believe that it is their fate to endure pain, to bite the bullet, to suffer in stoic silence. We disagree. Doctors have many effective ways of treating pain, and you should insist that your treatment plan include adequate pain control. More information on pain appears in chapter 13.

---

pleasant side effects, including swelling of tissues (edema), high blood pressure, diabetes, and ulcers.

Another group of drugs, the biophosphonates, prevents the breakdown of bone tissue that occurs when cancer metastasizes. Examples include clodronate, etidronate, and pamidronate.

Hot flashes, a common and unpleasant side effect of hormone therapy for prostate cancer, can be treated with megestrol acetate or clonidine.

Measuring the Impact of Drugs

A person's response to a drug is measured by improvements in various areas:

- Decrease in pain
- Increase in overall status (for example, an increase in energy)
- Stable or decreased PSA
- Weight stabilization
- Reduction in tumor burden (shrinking of tumor mass; fewer lesions on bone scan).

Judging by these standards, perhaps only one or two men out of ten who receive chemotherapy will get a little better. And any response may last for only a few months. Nor have studies shown that drugs will significantly lengthen survival time (Table 12.1).

Existing chemotherapy for prostate cancer poses a high risk of serious side effects, including nausea and vomiting, hair loss, lowered immunity, fatigue, weight loss, and damage to other organs such as the kidneys and liver. The slight benefits that might result from drug treatments for prostate cancer seldom outweigh the risks.

TABLE 12.1: RESPONSE TO EXPERIMENTAL DRUGS USED IN PROSTATE CANCER		
SINGLE DRUGS	**NUMBER OF STUDIES**	**COMPLETE OR PARTIAL RESPONSE**
5-FU	8	20%
Cisplatin	7	15%
Cyclophosphamide	5	5%
Doxorubicin	8	16%
Estracyt	12	5%
Hydroxyurea	3	22%
Methotrexate	1	5%
COMBINATION THERAPIES		
Cisplatin + doxorubicin	3	23%
Cyclophosphamide + doxorubicin	6	11%
Cyclophosphamide + doxorubicin + 5-FU	2	4%
Cyclophosphamide + methotrexate + 5-FU	2	11%
Doxorubicin + 5-FU + Mito-C	3	<1%

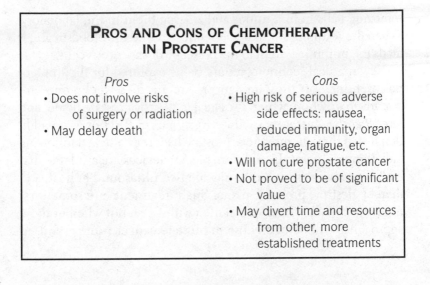

PROS AND CONS OF CHEMOTHERAPY IN PROSTATE CANCER

Pros	*Cons*
• Does not involve risks of surgery or radiation	• High risk of serious adverse side effects: nausea, reduced immunity, organ damage, fatigue, etc.
• May delay death	• Will not cure prostate cancer
	• Not proved to be of significant value
	• May divert time and resources from other, more established treatments

FUTURE DIRECTIONS: EXPERIMENTAL APPROACHES

New Therapies

Researchers are working to discover new approaches to prostate cancer treatment. Many of these experimental approaches are referred to as *biological therapies*, because they try to enlist the body's own systems to fight the disease.

Molecular biology involves changing cancer cells to make them more vulnerable to drugs or to the immune system. Some evidence suggests that a protein found in the prostate, called *uteroglobin*, interferes with the release of a substance that can cause cancer cells to spread. Altering that enzyme's activity may reduce the aggressiveness of a prostate tumor. Researchers are also investigating the use of *monoclonal antibodies*—molecules designed to seek out and destroy specific cells.

Immunotherapy attempts to defeat cancer in one of two main ways, either by stimulating the body's immune defenses to attack the cells directly or by causing cancer cells to become more vulnerable to an immune attack. One strategy now under study involves removing cells from a tumor and altering them in the laboratory. When the resulting substance is reinjected into the bloodstream, it alerts the immune system to the presence of cancerous cells.

New medical technologies are being explored for their potential usefulness in prostate cancer. Among these techniques are *electrovaporization*, which uses heat to destroy prostate tissue, and *laser therapy*, currently used for treatment of BPH or as an additional step for patients whose prostate becomes blocked following radiation treatment. In addition, several devices are available that use microwaves or high-intensity focused ultrasound to heat, and thereby destroy, prostatic tissue. Such treatments are sometimes used to reduce prostate size in men with BPH, but whether these approaches will be of any use in prostate cancer is uncertain. At

---

HOW TO ENROLL IN A DRUG STUDY

There are several ways patients and their physicians can learn about clinical trials. Specialists are likely to be aware of new experimental drugs in their field of practice and know which of their colleagues are conducting research. Participating hospitals frequently recruit volunteers through newspaper or radio ads explaining what kind of patients are wanted and how they can get further information about the study. If the idea of participating in a study interests you, talk to your physician.

Protecting the rights and safety of people who participate in drug testing is a major concern shared by drug sponsors, clinical investigators, and the Food and Drug Administration. The design of a clinical trial ensures that no participant will be subjected to unnecessary risk or be deprived of needed care merely to find out if a new drug is effective.

Those contemplating enrolling in a drug study should beware of quackery disguised as legitimate clinical research. To be sure you are volunteering for bona fide medical research, ask your doctor about the investigator, the institution, and the drug. If you decide to get in touch with the researchers, ask to see the informed-consent form, which explains the procedure and points out the risks. Insist on meeting with someone in authority who will explain the project to you in terms you can understand. Ask questions, and if you are not completely satisfied with the answers, do not agree to participate. Do not sign anything that waives your rights if you are harmed in the course of the study. No legitimate drug sponsor or investigator requires that.

Be very suspicious if you are asked to pay for an investigational drug. The FDA can allow drug sponsors to recover costs by selling investigational drugs, but only in the last stages of clinical trials and only when it is understood that the sponsor intends to bring the drug to market. This is not the usual pattern. Ask to see evidence that the FDA has approved both the study and the sale of the drug.

Be suspicious if you see the drug used in a "clinical trial" being advertised as effective treatment for people who have the disease. Such advertising violates FDA regulations. If you become aware of what appears to be health fraud masquerading as clinical research, call the nearest FDA office; it's listed in the phone book under United States Government.

—*Adapted from the American Cancer Society pamphlet*
"Questionable, Alternative, and Complementary Treatments
of Cancer: General Information," June 1995

this point none of these technological methods has proved to be effective in curing, or even controlling, prostate cancer.

Gene therapy involves introducing small but important sequences of DNA into a cell, causing the cell to act in a different way. As researchers decipher the complex code found in our DNA, more genetic approaches will inevitably be developed. At present, though, such therapy is years in the future.

Clinical Trials

Clinical trials are studies in which new treatments that showed some promise in laboratory experiments are tested in human volunteers. If you have an advanced stage cancer, or if your primary treatment did not result in a cure, you should consider taking part in a clinical trial. Keep in mind that just because a treatment is under study does not automatically mean it will be of value. That, after all, is what the trial is designed to find out. The treatment may not do any good; it may even make things worse. Nor should you think of participation in a clinical trial as a chance at a cure. At this time, there is no drug that will cure prostate cancer. On the other hand, by taking part in the trial, there is a chance you may experience some small benefit. If nothing else, your participation may help others. Negative results will tell us which treatments to avoid, and positive results will tell us which ones have a better chance of doing some good.

NONMEDICAL APPROACHES

Understandably, many people with a potentially life-threatening illness such as prostate cancer will do anything to get better. They'll grasp at any straw that promises to increase their chance of survival. If you base your choices on fear—fear of dying or fear of undergoing a risky, potentially painful treatment—you may be very vulnerable to false or misleading claims. Some of the people promoting these methods are well-meaning; others are unscrupulous and hope to exploit your fear for their own personal gain.

As doctors, we offer our patients only those treatments that have been subjected to years of rigorous, objective scientific study, usually first in animals and then in humans through clinical trials. We spend many hours each year carefully analyzing technical articles looking for evidence that a strategy will help relieve suffering. We are steadfastly committed to the scientific method and its objectivity. We also have faith in our nation's regulatory system, the Food and Drug Administration, which requires makers of drugs and medical devices to provide clear proof that their products indeed provide some benefit, to define the risks posed by their products, and to demonstrate that the benefits significantly outweigh the potential risks.

Our faith in conventional medical practice is not simply the product of bias. Here in the United States, established institutions, responsible practitioners, and conscientious pharmaceutical manufacturers that produce, test, and market new drugs and technologies are held to extremely high standards. Researchers who believe they have discovered something of value publish their results in journals; their findings are analyzed by other experts both before and after publication and tested again in subsequent studies. In other words, under our system, everyone plays by the same strict set of rules.

But for those who promote unconventional treatments, there are no rules. On one end of the "alternative treatment" spectrum we find the often highly publicized, too-good-to-be-true cancer "cures." The individuals and companies promoting these therapies often run their businesses in countries that lack the strict laws and government oversight found in the United States. They promote products whose contents are kept secret or technologies whose benefits are undocumented, let alone untested. If responsible people raise questions about these methods, the promoters respond that they are being victimized by a "conspiracy" of the so-called medical establishment to discredit them.

At the other end of the alternative spectrum are those who advocate such commonsense practices as eating a healthy diet, getting exercise, and learning how to manage stress. All of these methods can contribute to your general sense of well-being. By helping you stay focused on the joy of living, they can enhance your determination to get better. In many instances, those who promote lifestyle changes do not suggest that you abandon other, established forms of cancer treatment. However, no matter how much better alternative strategies make you feel, remember that these methods do not—cannot—directly address your basic problem: the dangerous cancerous growth inside your body, a cancer that will *never* disappear on its own.

Some argue that trying an alternative method "can't hurt." But certain unproven methods do indeed pose some very serious risks:

• They can divert time, money, and energy away from proven treatments.

• They can expose you to harmful chemicals, such as poisonous herbal compounds, or to dangerous techniques, such as whole-body hyperthermia. The American Cancer Society found, for example, that a "serum" used in an offshore cancer "clinic" was contaminated with the potentially lethal viruses that cause hepatitis and AIDS.

• They can interfere with proven treatments; for example, by rendering certain drugs ineffective.

• They can cause guilt, confusion, and frustration by putting you at odds with your doctors, family members, and others interested in your well-being.

• They can provide false hope.

We present the following information in the interest of completeness, to give you a full view of the range of approaches you will hear about as you explore your options. We make careful distinctions between those therapies that might confer some small benefit and those that are of highly questionable or negligible value. If you want additional information, contact organizations that research alternative therapies and that issue detailed reports on their findings, such as the American Cancer Society (1-800-ACS-2345) or the NCI/NIH Cancer Facts line (1-800-4-CANCER).

DIET

Dietary approaches are based on the premise that food can have a profound impact on the course of cancer. You should be aware that there is no scientific evidence to support this conclusion.

JUDGING CLAIMS

The American Cancer Society evaluates treatment methods by asking the following questions:

• Has the method been objectively demonstrated in the peer-reviewed scientific literature to be effective?

• Has the method shown potential for benefit that clearly exceeds the potential for harm?

• Have objective studies been correctly conducted under appropriate unbiased circumstances and subjected to peer-review scrutiny?

If you are trying to decide whether an alternative therapy is worth pursuing, you might ask the same questions of the people who are advocating it.

Three Dietary Strategies

There are three basic dietary strategies that people often use to fight cancer. The first, the "total nutritional approach," involves a radical restructuring of eating habits. One example is the macrobiotic diet, based on the Eastern principles of achieving balance between the two opposing forces of nature, yin and yang. Such a diet consists primarily of whole grains and beans. A person on a strict macrobiotic diet risks getting insufficient protein, vitamins, and minerals. Other nutritional therapies include the "wheatgrass" diet, which uses wheatgrass and other uncooked foods; various vegetarian diets (no meats; no animal products at all, including eggs or milk; etc.), and restricted diets alternating with occasional fasts.

A "special item diet" emphasizes one or more food items but does not necessarily involve a complete dietary overhaul. These diets come and go like the seasons. In recent years we've heard about the grapefruit diet, the popcorn diet, even the hard-boiled-egg diet.

The third main dietary strategy is the "supplemental approach," which calls for high doses of vitamins or minerals or the use of substances not normally found on the dinner table. Some people with prostate cancer make a point of consuming herbal teas, especially those containing essiac, echinacea, mistletoe extract, black cohosh, licorice, kelp, gotu kola, capsicum, ginger lobelia, or a substance called "pau d'arco." Recently a product called saw palmetto—an extract of berries from an American palm tree—has been used by some men with benign prostatic hyperplasia. Some people believe, without much evidence to back them up, that saw palmetto may be of use in prostate cancer.

Preliminary evidence suggests that modified citrus pectin, found in fruit fiber, may bind to the surface of metastasizing cancer cells and prevent them from "sticking" and forming tumors. Just eating a lot of oranges won't do the trick, because the pectin in fresh fruits is not absorbed by the body. Pectin has to be modified by a manufacturing process so that it will not be broken down during digestion.

Recently researchers found that men who eat higher amounts of cooked tomato products, such as tomato sauce, appeared to have a lower incidence of prostate cancer. Findings suggest that a substance in tomatoes, called lycopene, is responsible. These findings are provocative but not proved. Even if lycopene turns out to prevent prostate cancer, it would not necessarily follow that the substance would have any therapeutic effect on an established cancer.

A substance found in soybeans, genestein, may help block formation of blood vessels in a cancerous tumor.

Last, and perhaps least, is the "laetrile" of the 1990s: shark cartilage. Based on the misperception that sharks don't get cancer, some people concluded that eating shark cartilage would convey cancer immunity. So far, however, we have seen no proof that shark cartilage is of any benefit in preventing or treating prostate cancer.

Dietary Common Sense

There is no scientific evidence that dietary strategies affect prostate cancer to a significant degree. It is highly unlikely that eating certain foods or taking certain supplements will do much to control, let alone reverse, prostate cancer once it is present. We advocate a healthy diet that includes lots of fresh fruits and vegetables, whole grain foods, lots of fiber, a good mix of proteins, and low intake of fat. While it is known that by following these basic dietary guidelines you may lower your risk of several other types of cancer, there is no proof that following a "preventive" diet will do anything to stem cancer once it has developed.

Fat deserves some special discussion. Evidence strongly suggests that a high-fat diet contributes to the risk of prostate cancer. Studies have found that men who eat a lot of fat—five or more servings of red meat a week, for example—have a 79 percent higher risk of getting prostate cancer. Fat may somehow affect the surface of cells and make them more susceptible to cancerous growth. Since fat is also necessary for testosterone production, a diet high in fat may increase the supply of male hormones, which in turn fuels cancerous growth. The culprit appears to be an ingredient in fat called alpha-linolenic acid, found in red meat, whole milk products, butter, and processed soybean oil. The commonsense conclusion is that eating less fat could reduce the risk of prostate cancer. The other benefits that would accrue—weight reduction or a lower risk of heart disease, for example—make this a good idea overall.

Vitamins contain molecules your body uses to build and maintain healthy cells. Vitamins A, C, and E are classified as *antioxidants*, because they block the actions of certain oxygen molecules, known as *free radicals*, which can damage cell DNA and make the cell more likely to become cancerous. Vegetables that are dark green (for example broccoli, brussels sprouts, spinach) or dark yellow (carrots, squash, yams) contain high levels of antioxidants. Some of these vegetables contain beta-carotene, which the body converts into vitamin A. Good sources of vitamin C are citrus fruits, tomatoes, green peppers, and the dark green vegetables. Vitamin E comes from green leafy vegetables, whole grains, and vegetable oils.

Some research shows that the incidence of prostate cancer is higher in regions of the country that get less sunlight. Sunlight acts on chemicals in the skin to produce vitamin D, so it is possible that vitamin D plays a role in preventing prostate cancer. Dietary sources of vitamin D include sardines, fortified milk, and egg yolks.

A balanced diet will probably provide you with all the vitamins and minerals you need. If you feel you need additional amounts, don't rush out to your local health food store. Talk with a nutritionist first. Taking megadoses of some vitamins can be very dangerous. Besides, the body can hold only a certain amount of water-soluble vitamins, like vitamin C. Any excess is washed away. As one expert put it, "Some vitamin supplements do nothing but give you very expensive urine." Oil-soluble vitamins, such as A and E, can accumulate in the body and become toxic.

MIND-BODY THERAPIES

There are many other methods people with cancer have used in their quest for relief. Mind-body therapies are based on the premise that certain states of mind lead to better physical health. We will touch on a few of these methods here.

Biofeedback is a technique in which the person uses electrical monitors to develop a degree of conscious control over some of the body's automatic physical processes. Common uses of biofeedback include lowering blood pressure, altering pulse rate, and releasing muscle tension.

Meditation is focused concentration on an object or an idea to bring about an altered state of consciousness, usually deep relaxation or heightened awareness. Meditation may reduce stress, thus restoring the balance of body chemistry and helping the immune system function better.

Visualization is a technique in which the person focuses on mental images to trigger physical responses. One common strategy is to think of a pleasant scene and imagine that you are there enjoying the sights and sounds. Sometimes people visualize their bodies working to fight the cancer, imagining the cells of the immune system attacking the tumor, breaking it into pieces, and carrying it out of the body.

Acupuncture is a Chinese method in which needles are inserted into the skin to trigger physiological activity, such as the release of natural painkillers called endorphins.

Humor is a valuable tool in the fight against any illness. The men we know who are able to maintain their sense of humor despite their situation are the ones most likely to maintain their equilibrium and their zest for life.

Chapter 13

Recurring and Metastatic Cancer

Prostate cancer is stubborn. Years after treatment, there is a chance that the cancer may reemerge and new tumors may appear. Prostate cancer can also be aggressive. Many men don't find out they have it until it has already spread beyond the prostate gland.

A man whose cancer returns despite treatment faces different choices than does a man whose cancer is spreading. Both men, however, share the same goals: to manage the cancer, relieve any symptoms, and maintain the highest quality of life for as long as possible. Some men in those situations will continue to do well for years, even a decade or more. Others will not have as much time.

Your action plan is not complete unless you have taken into account all the possible scenarios—including the worst-case ones. There is no shame in feeling scared, but remember that much anxiety can arise just from feeling that recurring or metastatic cancer is making your life spin out of control. Knowing what to expect at this stage is a healthy way to gain some of that control.

CHANCES OF RECURRENCE AND METASTASIS

This chapter generally addresses high-stage cancer (stages T3 and T4 with metastases to one or more lymph nodes or distant sites). For a complete discussion of staging, see chapter 5. Here are some terms to keep in mind:

- *Recurring (or relapsing)*: describes cancer, regardless of its T stage, that returns after primary therapy

- *Refractory:* describes cancer that becomes unresponsive to hormonal treatment after a period of time
- *Metastasis:* spread of cancer to other places in the body
- *Clinical stage:* cancer stage as determined by diagnostic tests
- *Pathologic stage:* stage determined by direct evaluation of the tumor after radical prostatectomy

Even the most aggressive therapy given during the early stages does not always eliminate the cancer entirely or forever. The rate of *local recurrence* (return of cancer within the pelvis after treatment) is between 15 and 20 percent in men who have a radical prostatectomy and up to 28 percent in those who have external-beam radiation therapy. Seed implantation therapy and cryosurgery have not been around long enough to provide good statistics on how many men experience a return of their cancer. Generally, the higher the stage at diagnosis, the greater the risk of recurrence.

The development of metastases following recurrence of *early-stage* prostate cancer can take a long time—up to fifteen years in some cases. If your cancer is diagnosed at a later stage, though, the time before metastasis may be shorter.

In some cases the diagnostic workup finds metastases to one or more lymph nodes (stage N+) or to one or more distant sites (stage M+). Today, about one out of fifteen men who undergo radical prostatectomy are also found to have cancerous cells in the pelvic lymph nodes.

On hearing that their cancer has returned or spread, some men feel that they've been given a death sentence with no hope of reprieve. Worse, they feel that their remaining years will be marked by pain and suffering, not just from the disease but from the treatment. At this juncture, fear can become your worst enemy. You may be tempted to grasp at any therapeutic straw that promises even a modicum of relief. On the other hand, you may feel hopeless, that anything you do is futile, and you'll give up the fight entirely.

We believe that the best approach lies somewhere between these extremes. After you have absorbed the information in the pages that follow, go for a long walk. Talk things over with your spouse or partner, your children, your best buddy, and the doctor responsible for your care. You might also want to chat with a therapist and a member of the clergy. Contacting a support group is another possibility. Then decide for yourself what is most important to *you*. Design a plan that reflects your deepest desires and values.

The question you need to answer—and it's a tough one—is "How do I want to live the rest of my life?"

DETECTING RECURRENCE

Prostate cancer announces its return in any of several ways (see box). Elevated or rising PSA following treatment means there is a significant chance that the treatment has failed and that the prostate cancer has become active again, either locally or distantly. What constitutes an elevated PSA—and whether the degree of increase after curative therapy is significant—depends in large measure on the approach your doctor takes. Some define it as two consecutive elevations over a specific time period (two to six months, perhaps), while others take it to mean simply a steady rise after treatment. Ask your doctor to define this value for you early on. A diagnosis of recurrence means the time has come to implement the next phase of your treatment action plan.

In men who have not had radical prostatectomy, digital rectal examination can sometimes detect recurrence. Often rebiopsy reveals the presence of microscopic cancer, but even with a negative biopsy, there is still a greater than one in four chance that local recurrence will develop within ten years. A bone scan can reveal the presence of new lesions, which is why getting a baseline scan early on, before the cancer spreads, helps your doctor track its course later. Your doctor may also ask you to undergo tests for prostatic acid phosphatase (PAP) and alkaline phosphatase, and to rule out metastases to liver, lung, or lymph nodes.

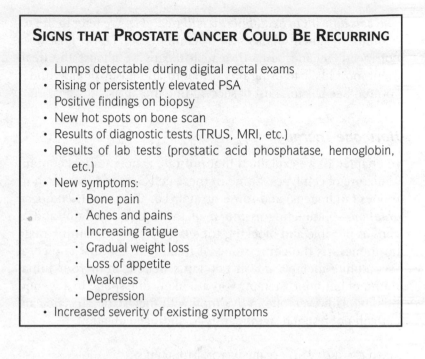

SIGNS THAT PROSTATE CANCER COULD BE RECURRING

- Lumps detectable during digital rectal exams
- Rising or persistently elevated PSA
- Positive findings on biopsy
- New hot spots on bone scan
- Results of diagnostic tests (TRUS, MRI, etc.)
- Results of lab tests (prostatic acid phosphatase, hemoglobin, etc.)
- New symptoms:
  - Bone pain
  - Aches and pains
  - Increasing fatigue
  - Gradual weight loss
  - Loss of appetite
  - Weakness
  - Depression
- Increased severity of existing symptoms

DNA ploidy tests may reveal more details about the exact nature of your tumor, which in turn may indicate your best treatment alternatives. According to one study, for example, *if* a patient's cancer involved one or more lymph nodes and *if* he had been treated aggressively with surgery and hormones, he stood a better chance of avoiding recurrence *if* his tumors happened to be diploid. That's a lot of "ifs," but such information may make a big difference in the treatment choices you have and their potential success.

TREATMENT CHOICES: SECOND-LINE THERAPY

The first line of defense against prostate cancer, of course, is aggressive therapy designed to bring about a cure. If the cancer recurs or spreads, you still have many options. *High-stage prostate cancer is difficult to treat, but it is still treatable.* We refer to the remaining treatment choices as "second-line therapy." That does not mean "second best." Instead it means we choose the treatment most likely to bring this stubborn and pushy disease under control. See box for a list of second-line therapies.

Hormone Therapy

In chapter 10 we explained that prostate cancer tumors contain a mixture of cell types. Some of these cells respond to male hormones (androgens) and some do not. For this reason, *androgen ablation*—eliminating as much of the body's supply of androgens as possible and blocking the effects of any remaining male hormones—is the cornerstone of treatment, the first choice of second-line therapy. If you got some benefit from your initial round of hormone therapy, you are likely to respond to a second helping. However, one in five men with metastatic prostate cancer will not respond significantly to androgen ablation.

SINGLE-AGENT AND COMBINATION THERAPIES
Some experts recommend the use of a single hormonal strategy (orchiectomy, LHRH agonist, or estrogen). Judging from the scientific evidence, each of these single agents is equally effective. Other experts advocate a combination of strategies, as discussed in chapter 10.

SECOND-LINE STRATEGIES

- Hormone therapy
- Chemotherapy
- Experimental strategies
- Salvage therapies
- Treatment for symptoms

OTHER DRUGS WITH HORMONAL EFFECTS

Tamoxifen, an agent commonly used in the treatment of breast cancer, is sometimes given to men with prostate cancer, either alone or in combination with other agents, and has produced some promising results. Investigators are studying other agents, including calcitonin, spironolactone, and diphosphonates, but results so far are not encouraging.

WHY NOT SURGERY?

If removing the testicles works by eliminating most of the androgen supply, it would seem logical to remove other tissues involved in androgen production. However, surgery to remove the adrenal glands (*adrenalectomy*) or to incapacitate the pituitary gland (*hypophysectomy*) has only limited impact on progressing prostate cancer. The risks of these procedures are unacceptably high; besides, most of the same benefits can be achieved with medication. For these reasons, surgical approaches are rarely, if ever, used today (except as discussed on p. 200).

TIMING OF HORMONE THERAPY

With hormone therapy the question is not just which strategy to use, but when. You may feel it is important to do everything possible immediately. Or you may prefer to take a "wait and see" approach. Whichever you choose, there is evidence to support your decision.

One strategy is to begin hormone therapy as soon as the cancer recurs and to continue indefinitely. If you elect not to have an orchiectomy, it is probably best to plan on continuing use of an LHRH agonist.

Another strategy is to delay treatment until symptoms appear, such as bone pain or bladder outlet obstruction. Hormones can often do a lot to relieve pain.

With hormone therapy, PSA levels may return to normal, the primary tumor may shrink, and metastases may decrease in size

HORMONE THERAPY AS A STRATEGY

- Single agent
  - Orchiectomy
  - LHRH agonist (e.g., leuprolide, goserelin)
  - Estrogen
  - Progestin
- Combination therapy
- Other drugs with hormonal effects
  - Tamoxifen
  - Calcitonin, etc.
- Surgical strategies (very rarely used)
  - Adrenalectomy
  - Hypophysectomy
- Timing of therapy
  - Immediate
  - Delayed
  - Continuous
  - Intermittent
- Medical suppression of adrenal glands (see chapter 10)
  - Ketoconazole
  - Liarozole

and number. Some experts argue that treatment should stop when relapse occurs, since the cells that are not responding to hormones have become the majority population. Others point out that tumors contain a mixture of cells, and that hormone therapy should be continued even though it keeps only the androgen-dependent cells at bay.

WHICH WAY TO GO?
We wish we could sift through the piles of medical literature and grab the one article that states conclusively, once and for all, which hormone strategy you or any other man should adopt for recurring or metastatic cancer. Unfortunately, no such article exists.

Instead you might want to consider the results of a survey conducted a few years ago at Memorial Sloan-Kettering Cancer Center in New York. Researchers compared the quality of life of two groups of patients: those who elected to receive hormone therapy (either DES or LHRH plus flutamide) as soon as metastatic prostate cancer was diagnosed, and those who decided to wait. The patients filled out a questionnaire with forty-nine items covering physical complaints (fatigue, pain, urinary problems, hot flashes, loss of appetite, nausea and vomiting, sleep deprivation, breast enlargement), sexual problems (interest level, enjoyment, ability to get an erection), psychological distress, interference with family or social life, intrusive thoughts regarding cancer, and marital communication problems. They filled out the questionnaire a month after the study started, and again at the two-month and six-month marks.

The results were somewhat surprising. The men who decided *not* to have therapy had a higher overall quality of life than those taking hormones. They reported fewer sexual problems and more physical energy. After six months, they actually experienced a drop in their level of psychological distress. In contrast, the men on hormones reported a *rise* in distress. Perhaps the rise was due to the fact that hormone treatments caused adverse effects; perhaps it was because they were being constantly reminded of their illness—and their mortality—by taking daily pills or visiting the doctor for monthly shots; or maybe it was simply because the men who deferred therapy were less concerned about how many days they had left and were more focused on living fully from day to day.

Chemotherapy

If you have recurring cancer, chemotherapy may be an option for you. Drugs cannot cure prostate cancer, and they may not add significantly to survival, but in some cases they can help to control the cancer and relieve symptoms. The chemotherapy strategies described in chapter 12 are the same ones that are used for recurring prostate cancer.

Drugs used singly include many of the standard anticancer agents: adriamycin, mitoxantrone, cyclophosphamide, vinblastine, and 5-fluorouracil (5-FU). Recently, scientists have become interested in the use of mitomycin C, among the most potent cancer-cell killers yet identified. One study found that about 30 percent of men with high-stage prostate cancer showed at least a partial response to this agent.

These drugs are usually used in combination. Promising strategies include cis-platinum plus etoposide and methotrexate plus buserelin. A recent study of taxol plus estramustine found that one in three men showed a significant decline in PSA level, lasting about seven months. Estramustine plus etoposide may be helpful in *small-cell cancer,* a rare form of prostate cancer that usually doesn't respond to hormone therapy. More than half of the men given this regimen showed a drop in PSA of 50 percent or more, and one in three had other signs of improvement.

Salvage Therapies

Under certain circumstances it may be possible to use first-line therapies as second-line treatments against recurring prostate cancer. As the term *salvage* suggests, these methods are attempts to make the best of a difficult situation.

SALVAGE SURGERY AFTER RADIATION

A high PSA level or a rising PSA a year after radiation therapy is a sign that the disease is still active. Positive biopsy after treatment confirms it. In such cases, radical prostatectomy might be considered. To be eligible, you should be in otherwise good health and highly motivated to undergo another significant therapy. You should also have a negative bone scan and CT or MRI scan to make sure the cancer has not spread. Surgery after radiation therapy has a very high risk of adverse effects. The rate of incontinence is between 5 and 30 percent, and the risk of impotence is nearly 100 percent. Damage to the bladder or rectum occurs in up to 16 percent of men. Other risks include damage to the ureters, blood loss, and death.

Cryosurgery may also be attempted following radiation therapy, but studies have not yet demonstrated whether this approach has any value, and it does carry significant risks.

SALVAGE RADIATION

Radiation is sometimes given following radical prostatectomy if the surgical margins are positive or if there is a rising PSA but no signs that the cancer has spread beyond the pelvis (stage T3, N+, M0). The dose is typically lower than when radiation is given as first-line treatment because, with the prostate gland gone, there is less of a target. Deferring salvage radiation until the PSA rises may be too late; for that reason, some experts recommend radiation therapy at or near the time of radical prostatectomy. Some investigators found that 45 percent of men treated with salvage radiation were cancer-free for five years.

Radiation oncologists perform radiation seed implantation following external-beam radiation in some men. Such an approach can result in good control of the tumor, but there is no evidence yet that it increases survival, and it does involve significant risks.

A second course of external-beam radiation may be given, but such instances are very rare.

SALVAGE ANDROGEN THERAPY

Physicians are investigating the effectiveness of DES at the time of radiation for stage T3 cancers. Early evidence suggests that this technique may not reduce local recurrence, but it may prevent metastases.

Symptomatic Treatment

If recurring or metastatic cancer progresses to the point at which it causes symptoms, the focus needs to shift away from treating the cancer and toward dealing with your life as a whole.

PAIN CONTROL

The single most important priority of care at this phase is the relief of pain. Pain is cancer's cruel accomplice. A constant reminder that something is wrong, pain saps your energy, impairs your functioning, and interferes with treatment. Over time it can interfere with your ability to eat, to digest, to walk, to think. Pain must be treated, and treated aggressively.

Many men in our culture were brought up to believe that if they want to be a "man," they have to endure pain. Think of the slogans athletes live by: "No pain, no gain." "Play through the pain." "Take it like a man." Often, men refuse to admit, acknowledge, or express pain for fear they'll be considered a "sissy," a "crybaby," a "whiner," a "wimp."

On the other hand, some studies have found that sometimes doctors may not do enough to relieve pain.

There is no need to suffer from the pain of prostate cancer. You should be as assertive about getting pain relief as you are about the other aspects of your treatment. Effective therapy is available, but if you do not acknowledge your pain and tell your doctor about it, you cannot get the help you need.

Evaluation: The first step is learning to talk to your doctor about pain. Try to describe it accurately: Where does it strike? Under what conditions? How long does it last? Does anything help make it go away? What does the pain feel like—stabbing, throbbing, burning, dull? If possible, make notes about your pain and bring them to your appointments.

Most pain from advanced prostate cancer comes from metastases to the bone. Over time, cancer cells replace bone cells, weakening their structure and crowding other tissues. If the metastases are lodged in the spinal column, there is danger that the vertebrae will start to compress. This may put pressure on the nerves and the spinal cord, which produces even more pain and could lead to paralysis. Your doctor will first determine if this is the cause, since pain from this source requires a special treatment approach.

Treatment with Radiation: Radiation is one of the two basic approaches to pain management in prostate cancer (the other is drugs). *External-beam radiation,* usually given in conjunction with a hormonal pain reliever such as dexamethasone, is essential for treating spinal cord compression. It is also used for pain arising from individual metastases at other sites, including the liver, brain, and chest cavity. A typical course of radiation treatment is 2,000 to 3,000 cGy given over a two- or three-week period—about a third of the dosage used for treating the cancer itself. Results can be dramatic. Between 80 and 90 percent of men experience a significant improvement, and more than half will enjoy complete relief. One drawback is that radiation sometimes limits the use of other systemic palliative treatments for prostate cancer. That's because it can deplete the supply of bone marrow, the chief source of blood cells including the white cells that are part of the immune system. People with low white-cell counts are more vulnerable to infections.

Recently, some treatment centers have begun treating widespread metastases using a technique called *half-body radiation,* in which the beam is applied to large areas of the body rather than to a few select sites. About two thirds of men who receive treatment to the lower body and 82 percent of those treated in the upper body will have relief from pain for as long as they live.

Treatment with Medications: The Ladder Strategy: Typically the strategy for use of pain medications is to begin with the simplest treatment and step up the attack if and when necessary. Pain experts refer to this as the *ladder* approach.

On the first rung of the ladder are acetaminophen and the nonsteroidal anti-inflammatory agents—aspirin and ibuprofen, and its cousins. These can be surprisingly effective. If more relief is needed, nonsteroidals containing pain-killing agents called *opioids* are brought into play. Examples include ketoprofen and ketorolac. One drawback of these medications is that there is a limit to their effectiveness. If the pain increases, taking more of the drug won't do any further good.

The next step is to use *narcotic agents* such as morphine. The fact that pain is so often undertreated in this country has much to do with the myths and misunderstandings people have about narcotics, especially the fear of addiction. *Addiction* is the continued use of a drug for purposes other than medical treatment. It is also the inability to stop using the drug despite clear evidence that it is causing harm (physical, emotional, and financial) to the addict and the addict's family. People who use narcotics for their intended purpose—pain relief—are not addicts. Moreover, the chance that they'll become addicted is low. Once the pain stops, so does their use of the medication. Over time, the body may develop a *tolerance* to narcotics. This means that progressively higher doses are needed to achieve the same degree of relief. Tolerance is *not* the same as addiction.

Pain control is an essential part of the management of advanced prostate cancer. Fear of addiction is no excuse for your doctor to withhold narcotic treatments, or for you to resist taking them.

Recently the use of medications containing *radioactive isotopes* has added another rung to the pain control ladder. The best known of these is Metastron, which contains strontium. This drug is given in a single injection that provides pain relief lasting up to six months. Repeat injections are possible. About 20 percent of men will enjoy total relief, and another 60 percent or so will experience at least partial relief. There are few side effects—the most common is flushing (redness and heat)—and, unlike narcotics, Metastron does not cause nausea, vomiting, or constipation. Other isotopes are also under study. These treatments don't work quickly or strongly enough to prevent pain from spinal cord compression.

Other Strategies: A number of nonmedical treatments may provide a significant level of pain relief. Among these are relaxation techniques, biofeedback, self-hypnosis, yoga, and meditation. Some caregivers recommend use of TENS (transcutaneous electronic nerve stimulation), an electronic device that delivers a mild electric current to the nerves and activates the body's natural painkilling systems.

Talk with your doctor about which of these might be appropriate for you. And be aware that metastases can weaken your bones, especially bones of the arms and legs. To reduce risk of fractures or breaks, you should not exercise until you have been evaluated.

RELIEVING OTHER SYMPTOMS

Pain usually requires the most aggressive treatment, but it is not the only symptom of advanced prostate cancer. Some men experience a syndrome known as *cachexia*, involving loss of appetite, weight loss, muscle wasting, and overall fatigue. Use of prednisone or megestrol acetate, either in short intermittent courses or in long-term administration, can relieve these symptoms and increase the sense of well-being.

If lymph nodes become clogged with cancerous cells or their byproducts, they can obstruct veins and lead to circulation problems. Hormone treatment may help.

In some cases urinary symptoms—frequency, urgency, obstruction—may become serious enough to warrant attention. A man who has not had a prostatectomy may benefit from a transurethral resection of the prostate.

COMING TO TERMS WITH DEATH

No matter how complete your action plan is, or how thorough your caregivers are, or how supportive your loved ones have been, there may come a time when you must accept the fact that you have a terminal disease. About 80 percent of men with prostate cancer that has metastasized to bone (stage M+) will die within five years, regardless of the treatment they receive. That very unpredictability is both a curse and a blessing: A curse, because uncertainty breeds anxiety and fear; a blessing, because every new day is another opportunity for joy, for fulfillment . . . for discovering what it truly means to be alive.

Give some thought to what makes your life worth living. You'll find it easier to handle tough choices if you come to terms with your cancer, set your priorities, and make the most of the time ahead.

Make sure your will is complete and up to date. Get all your paperwork in order: deeds, insurance plans, trusts. If you have specific feelings about medical treatments, discuss them with your family and your doctor. Have a *living will* on file that spells out which medical therapies you will not accept should you become incapacitated or are unable to make decisions. Consult a lawyer about signing forms that give others the authority to make decisions on your behalf (known as "durable power of attorney"). Just as important, be sure the people you put in this position know what your specific choices are and are willing to see that they are carried out.

Take care of unfinished business. Visit places you've always wanted to see, do things you've always wanted to do. Even if you can't conquer Mt. Everest or win the decathlon, you can still savor a hot dog at the ballpark, or take your granddaughter for an afternoon at the zoo, or sit with your arm around your wife as you watch the sunrise over a misty lake. Most important, tell the people you love how you feel about them.

An ancient Japanese story seems pertinent here. A Buddhist monk walking along a mountain trail trips on a stone and tumbles over a cliff. As he falls he manages to grab a root sticking out from the cliffside. Now dangling in the air, he looks up and sees a mouse nibbling away at the root. Looking down he sees a hungry tiger pacing below, waiting for him to fall. Just then he notices a wild strawberry growing on the side of the cliff. He reaches for it and pops it into his mouth. *How sweet it tastes!*

VOICES OF EXPERIENCE

After learning that his prostate cancer had reached stage T4, Bill, a sixty-year-old retail sales manager from California, had some choices to make. "I studied a hell of a lot. My experience as a manager taught me that if you have a solution available, you'd better use it now because you may not get a chance later." He and his doctors agreed on an aggressive course of treatment: first hormone therapy, then surgery, then radiation. "I'm glad I knew the dangers in advance, because everything that could go wrong with my treatment did go wrong. But I was prepared. Even the risk of death has been easier to handle, because I knew it was a possibility from the start. I know the cancer may kill me sooner or later, but at least I feel comfortable knowing I've made the most of the time given to me."

By the time Carl, age seventy-four, found out he had prostate cancer, it had already metastasized to the bones in his hips. A former fighter pilot in World War II and at the time a retired airline executive, he later confided to his wife, "Never in my life did I feel as hopeless and frightened as the day I got that diagnosis." Somehow, though, Carl was able to convert his fear into action. With hormone therapy keeping the cancer in check, and radiation therapy controlling the pain, Carl spent the next few months calling old friends, visiting with his children and grandchildren, even planning his own memorial service. "I want this to be the biggest damned party anyone ever saw," he said. Those who attended the service—held, fittingly, in an airline hangar—agreed that it was.

Chapter 14

Incontinence

For many men, the most worrisome potential problem following treatment for prostate cancer is incontinence: the inability to control urine. Incontinence is a throwback to infancy, when we could not control our bodies, and the association triggers feelings of helplessness, dependency, sadness, and fear. Often men find it easier to accept loss of their erections, or to confront their mortality, than to imagine themselves wearing diapers or having a urine-collection bag strapped to their leg.

Normally we don't think about it, but urine control is a twenty-four-hour-a-day job. That's why the impact of incontinence on lifestyle can be enormous. The thought that throwing a bowling ball or swinging a golf club or doing a Texas two-step might make him spring a leak, or that he might be emitting an offensive odor, is enough to keep many a man home on Saturday night. Getting up many times at night—or worse, not getting up in time—can make it impossible for a man and his wife to get a decent night's sleep.

Fortunately, permanent incontinence following prostate cancer treatment is rare. While some level of urinary complication may occur, there is a lot that can be done to manage the situation, even before treatment starts. For most men, the problem will improve dramatically over time—usually weeks or months—and their lives will return to normal.

WHY IT HAPPENS

The prostate's location is what makes incontinence such a problem. Remember that the urethra is the tube carrying urine from the bladder through the prostate and through the penis. Just outside the prostate, the urethra is surrounded by the sphincter muscles, which are responsible for keeping the tube closed. When a man urinates, the muscles relax; when he's finished, they tighten up again.

Removing the prostate surgically inevitably means cutting out the part of the urethra passing through the prostate. It also may mean removal of part of the sphincter muscles. Depending on how extensive the tumor is, the surgeon may remove tissue at the bladder neck which adjoins the prostate. The bladder neck is a ring of muscles that act as shut-off valves, and these muscles extend down to form part of the urethra. After the prostate is out, the surgeon reattaches the bladder to the urethra. Even if the job is done correctly, with meticulous placement of the sutures, there may be strain on or damage to these muscles, and leakage can result.

Radiation is usually less likely to cause incontinence, but both external-beam therapy and seed implantation can damage tissues. If scarring results, the muscles lose some of their ability to control urine flow.

Although cryosurgery does not involve cutting, it too poses a risk of incontinence because there is a danger that part of the urethra or nearby bladder tissue can be frozen and damaged.

Sometimes prostate cancer treatment can cause urinary voiding symptoms, such as frequency (the need to urinate often) or urgency (the inability to delay urination once the feeling strikes). What we're talking about in this chapter, though, is the inability to contain urine.

RISK

It is difficult to quantify what the precise risk of incontinence following prostate cancer treatment is. Some confusion arises because different people define the problem differently. For some men, incontinence means not being completely dry and in control 100 percent of the time. Others feel that having to use a small pad or two each day to absorb any stray droplets or having to wear absorbent pads only at night qualifies as "continence."

Another factor in the equation is time. Nearly everyone is incontinent for a period of time after prostate surgery. The question is, how long will the problem last? Some men regain control within days after the catheter is removed. Others take longer, often many months. We know of cases in which full continence hadn't returned for a year—but it did return. So the answer to the question, "Do you have a problem with incontinence?" may very well depend on how much time has elapsed.

Individual circumstances come into play. Incontinence is a problem often associated with aging, even in otherwise healthy men. The older you are, the greater your risk.

One last point: Many studies on incontinence are done as surveys, which basically means researchers ask patients if they're having any problems. Often men are reluctant to complain about what they might feel is a minor nuisance, or they don't want to risk offending their caregivers by suggesting they could have done a better job. Or they may be too embarrassed to talk about it.

The statistic you'll hear cited most often is that, overall, up to 3 percent of men are incontinent a year after treatment. That figure, however, represents the number of men who may never regain full urinary control. Another 10 to 15 percent may continue to experience varying degrees or types of urinary problems such as stress incontinence (losing urine only during times of physical stress, such as sneezing or coughing). The remaining group of men includes those who are completely continent as well as those who have "occasional" spotting. Again, for many of these men, control will continue to improve over time.

How long will the problem persist? That, too, is hard to predict. If you're the one who's incontinent, any time is too long. Still, there is usually light at the end of the tunnel. "It took nine months for me to get straightened out," commented Art, a sixty-six-year-old shock trauma technician from Colorado Springs. "I was in diapers for a while. Finally shed those, but then wasn't able to void, so I needed a catheter. Eventually the doctors discovered they needed to stretch my urethra, so they did that procedure once a week for four weeks. But by nine months after my radical prostatectomy, I was completely dry, and I've stayed that way for the last five years." In contrast, Ken, a seventy-two-year-old retired journalist from South Carolina, had nearly regained full control by the time he was discharged from the hospital. "My wife had already bought me a supply of adult diapers," he said, "but we were delighted to make the trip to the store and get our money back."

TYPES OF INCONTINENCE

Stress incontinence involves loss of urine during exercise or sudden movement. Normally, the sphincter muscles are strong enough to keep the floodgates closed. A little extra pressure, however—standing up after sitting in a chair, or swinging a three-iron—and leakage can occur.

Urge incontinence is the result of involuntary bladder contractions. Normally the bladder is controlled by part of the brain that determines when conditions are right for urinating. With urge incontinence, the bladder simply decides to start emptying "without permission." Men with urge incontinence begin to leak urine with little or no provocation or warning. For some, the problem arises if they think about going to the bathroom, or if they hear or touch running water. Urge incontinence causes annoyingly frequent and rushed trips to the men's room.

Overflow incontinence involves the nearly continuous loss of small amounts of urine throughout the day and at night. This results from having a full bladder that is incapable of emptying completely, either because flow is obstructed or because the nerve supply to the bladder is faulty. In some cases overflow incontinence is associated with a sensation of incomplete bladder emptying.

TREATMENTS

To an extent, dealing with incontinence is like dealing with prostate cancer itself: If a cure is possible, we go for it. If not, then we try to manage the situation to provide the best possible quality of life.

Your choice of treatment depends on the exact nature of your problem. Here are some of the options.

Behavioral Techniques

A behavioral technique involves learning a new pattern of action. These methods are easy, cheap, and remarkably effective. Behavioral methods alone can produce significant improvement in most cases and may even be enough in themselves to end the problem.

KEGEL EXERCISES

One of the simplest methods for strengthening the pelvic muscles is the Kegel exercise. Named for the physician who developed them, Kegel exercises (or "Kegels") work the same as any conditioning method: by flexing and relaxing a muscle, you build up tone and stamina. Doing Kegels regularly is probably the single most effective step you can take to regain urinary control. If you happen to be reading this before your therapy for prostate cancer begins, you might want to ask your doctor whether you should start doing Kegels now.

You already do Kegels, but you might not have known that they had a name. A Kegel is that squeezing maneuver you make at the end of urinating, a tightening up of the buttocks and anus. To get a real sense of the Kegel exercise, the next time you're urinating, stop the flow midstream and count to three. Those are the muscles involved. For continence training, Kegels can be done at your convenience at one or more times during the day (see box). Check with your doctor before doing Kegels.

KEGEL EXERCISES

Here's the Kegel exercise routine as developed at Beth Israel Hospital in Boston:
- While standing, squeeze the pelvic muscles and hold for up to ten seconds. Remember to breathe while squeezing. It may help to count out loud.
- Relax for a count of ten.
- Repeat as often as you can, up to fifteen times, until you are tired or unable to keep squeezing for the full ten seconds.
- Relax for a minute or so.
- Do a short-cycle exercise: Squeeze for one second, then relax for a second. Repeat that ten times, then rest for a moment.
- Repeat the short-cycle pattern ten times.
- Do the exercises as often as your doctor allows.

Exercise only the pelvic muscles. There's no benefit in tensing up other muscles during this routine.

BLADDER TRAINING

There are several methods for conditioning the bladder which can be useful for those who experience either stress incontinence or urge incontinence.

Prompted voiding is a fancy term for "peeing on a schedule." If you can tell your bladder to release urine on the schedule you dictate, you are on your way to controlling incontinence. At first, try going to the bathroom once an hour, whether you feel the urge or not. Gradually lengthen the time between visits. Eventually your bladder should get the message.

You might want to consider biofeedback or electrical stimulation as a strategy for bladder training. These methods use devices that help you recognize when you're doing things correctly. Once you get used to the feelings, you can take the same steps on your own. Ask your urologist whether such methods are right for you.

PREVENTIVE STEPS FOR INCONTINENCE

• Watch what you eat and drink. Certain foods have diuretic properties: That means they draw water out of your body tissues more quickly and thus generate more urine. Examples include caffeinated drinks (coffee, tea, cola) and alcohol. Chocolate and certain medications also contain caffeine. Cut back on the amount of liquid you take in. Whenever possible, drink only water. Check with your doctor, and perhaps a nutritionist, to make sure you are getting just enough of the right kinds of liquid to stay healthy.

• Lose weight. In men, excess body fat tends to accumulate in the abdomen, where it pushes down on the bladder. This in turn increases the degree of sphincter muscle tone required to keep the urine where it belongs. Talk to your doctor to see if weight reduction is okay for you.

• If you feel a sneeze or a cough coming on, cross your legs and do a Kegel.

• Try to keep your bladder empty, especially at bedtime or before engaging in a vigorous activity.

• Wear protective pads or undergarments.

• Deal with "after-dribble." The male urethra is somewhat like the plumbing under a sink: There's a curve in the pipe where urine can collect. Men coping with incontinence may need to be a little more aware of the need to drain the leftover urine from the penis before zipping up.

ANTICIPATORY MANAGEMENT

Just as you know the right moment to reach for a tissue when you feel a sneeze coming on, you can also take steps to anticipate—and prevent—urinary accidents. Some of these are listed in the box above.

Urine Control Products

USEFUL METHODS

In those cases in which occasional dribble is the extent of the problem, many men manage by inserting a pad or a folded paper towel between the penis and the undergarment. Some go an extra step by wearing underpants with a specially designed absorbent pouch. The pouch surrounds the penis and catches leaks, but it doesn't extend below and behind your scrotum, so it doesn't cause irritation. These garments come in different sizes with different fluid capacities, depending on the severity of the problem.

If these are inadequate, adult diapers are an option. If you find the notion of wearing a diaper unthinkable, try to remind yourself that, in most instances, the problem will diminish with time. It can also help to join a support group to vent feelings and frustrations, to learn how others cope, and—most important—to realize that you are not alone in this struggle (see chapter 16).

QUESTIONABLE METHODS

A few urine control methods may do more harm than good if they prevent you from doing the muscle and bladder conditioning you need to return to full continence.

One such device is a special clamp that fastens tightly around the penis and obstructs the flow. Besides being counterproductive in the long haul, this device poses some short-term risks. Left on too long, it can impair blood flow, damaging the penile skin or even the urethral channel deep inside. If the clamp is used at all, it should be for only a short time (no more than a few hours) and should not be used at all during the first two months of recovery. Ideally, it should be removed every hour or so to allow urine to pass. Otherwise urine can build up; the feeling can be unpleasant, like trying to stop urinating in midstream.

Another of the less-desirable options in the early recovery period is the condom catheter, a sheath that fits over the penis and allows urine to drain through a tube into a bag attached to the leg.

Again, such a device can possibly work against your efforts at early recovery. If you never have to worry about controlling your urine, you won't be motivated to do your exercises and you may not regain control as quickly. That said, the condom catheter is a reasonable choice when other methods fail and leakage is severe or permanent.

Medications

Certain medications can contribute to restoring some level of bladder and sphincter control. If you develop an infection in the urinary tract, inflammation can irritate the system and trigger the unwanted release of urine. Antibiotics can alleviate the problem.

Men who experience stress incontinence sometimes improve while taking drugs that increase sphincter muscle tone. Physicians sometimes prescribe phenylpropanolamine (which is also available in over-the-counter preparations) to help restore tone to the urethral muscles.

Urge incontinence has been treated successfully with anticholinergic drugs, which act on the nervous system to alleviate involuntary bladder spasms. Such medications as Ditropan, Pro-Banthine, Levsin, and Tofranil are anticholinergic drugs, as are many of the prescription-strength cough suppressants.

Medication usually produces favorable results. By some estimates, three of four men show at least some improvement. For a minority of men, medications plus muscle conditioning exercises may be all they need to keep the incontinence under control. These medications, as expected, can produce unwanted side effects. If one medication disagrees with you, your physician may be able to switch you to a different one that you tolerate better.

Surgical Procedures

Sometimes treatment for prostate cancer can result in a *stricture*, a narrowing of the urethra or the bladder neck that results when scar tissue forms. In most cases, stricture can be managed through a simple procedure called *urethral dilation*, performed in the urologist's office under a local anesthetic or sedation. First, the physician inspects your urethra using a cystoscope, a telescopic viewing instrument. When the stricture is found, slender tubes of gradually increasing size are inserted to gently press the scar tissue back. If the problem is not resolved the first time, the procedure may be repeated. Another alternative is to surgically cut the stricture, using special telescopic instruments or a beam of laser light. In most cases these steps will take care of the problem.

In rare instances, if severe incontinence persists for longer than a year, an artificial sphincter may be the answer. This is a silicone device that has an inflatable cuff that wraps around the urethra. The device is implanted inside the body. When inflated, the cuff squeezes the urethra shut. When you need to urinate, you deflate the cuff (the valve is tucked inside the scrotum). The pump automatically reinflates after a few minutes, again blocking urine flow. An artificial sphincter, placed by a surgeon with experience in the procedure, is the best option for men with serious persistent incontinence; it can often produce a dramatic improvement in the quality of life.

Implanting the artificial sphincter is a relatively costly surgical procedure requiring the use of anesthesia and hospitalization. Adverse effects may include bleeding, infection, and a problem releasing urine at the right time (urinary retention). In rare cases, the device can malfunction or break, requiring reoperation. Sometimes the seal provided by the cuff is incomplete, causing a minor leakage of urine.

A few years ago, the FDA approved *collagen injections* as a new method of treating incontinence (Fig. 14.1). Collagen is a fibrous molecule that occurs naturally in the body and that makes up about 90 percent of your skin. Injected into the tissue surrounding the urethra, collagen adds "bulk" to the region and helps the urethra to close. The procedure, which takes about thirty min-

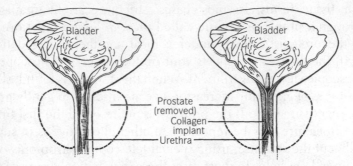

***Figure 14.1: Collagen implants to restore
the function of the urethra.***

utes, can be done on an outpatient basis under local or general
anesthesia or sedation. Using a cystoscope, the surgeon guides the
needle to the desired site and injects the collagen. A skin test is
given several weeks before the first procedure to make sure the
patient is not allergic to the substance.

The procedure has its drawbacks. The body can reabsorb part
of the injected material, thereby reducing the bulking effect and
requiring reinjection—in some cases as many as five or more
times. Collagen implants have not been in use very long. Some
studies suggest that between one third and one half of men who
have them notice improved or complete bladder control.
Whether the implants will remain effective over long periods is
not yet known.

VOICES OF EXPERIENCE

We'll give the last word on incontinence to Arnold, age sixty-five,
an advertising executive in Connecticut:

"My doctor warned me to be prepared to work for a year at re-
gaining control. He was right. I worked at my exercises diligently,
and there were times when I felt I took two steps forward and one

or two back. In my worst moments I thought I would wear a diaper forever, and I felt pretty down. The overall trend, though, was positive. Over the course of several months I progressed from a diaper to a smaller pad and finally a mini-pad. It took the better part of a year to feel comfortable enough not to use anything for protection. For a while I had leaking sensations, but when I checked myself I would be dry. I consider myself a hundred percent dry now, although on occasion—if I've had a lot of caffeine or am tired—I may lose a drop or two.

"The bottom line is, don't give up, keep up the exercises, get back to a normal life as fast as you can, and keep yourself physically fit. I am a firm believer that mental attitude and physical fitness can work wonders on your recovery."

Chapter 15

Impotence

If you're worried about becoming impotent as a result of prostate cancer and its treatment, here is good news: *You can get your erections back.* You may have to learn a few new tricks—and you and your partner may have to rediscover what true intimacy is all about—but even after cancer treatment you can still enjoy a full and satisfying sex life.

Unfortunately, the word *impotence* is misleading and inaccurate. The term literally means "lack of power," and it's that image of powerlessness and humiliation that triggers fear and anxiety in men. In its broadest clinical meaning, though, impotence simply means a problem achieving or maintaining a good erection. Many caregivers prefer to use the term *erectile dysfunction*. That's not just medical jargon; it's a more accurate statement of the problem.

Perhaps the biggest misconception is that if you're impotent, you can't experience orgasm. An impotent man's penis is virtually as sensitive and tender as before. *You don't have to have an erection to have an orgasm.* The sex organ most responsible for orgasm is located not between your legs but above your neck: your brain. The brain is responsible for sexual interest, arousal, and the sensations you experience, along with the emotions you feel that make sex worthwhile: love, tenderness, and affection. Another myth is that you must be able to ejaculate fluid to experience orgasm. Removal of the prostate, the seminal vesicles, and the testicles takes away the sources of semen but does not eliminate the pleasurable feeling. This is why you don't need an erection or a prostate to have an orgasm — just a penis and a brain. An erection is necessary for penetration, though, and modern medicine offers methods to help almost every man in this regard.

No matter what treatment you choose for prostate cancer, you can still be powerful, passionate, and sexy.

In this chapter we'll describe the many ways available to deal with impotence. You'll probably need some help in choosing the method that's right for you. Plan now to involve your partner in the decision, because, after all, you're not the only one affected. Think deeply about what having sex really means and how important it is to both of you. If you and your mate have sex a few times a year, you will probably choose a different impotence treatment than will a couple who is more sexually active. For additional guidance on coping with prostate cancer and its consequences as a couple, see chapter 16.

ANATOMY

To understand impotence and its remedies, it helps to have a clear idea of how your sex organs work. You might want to take another look at chapter 2 for a more detailed discussion.

Erections are the product of a well-engineered hydraulic system. When you become sexually aroused, the nerves that travel near the prostate gland signal arteries to increase the blood flow into the three chambers of the penis (the two *corpora cavernosa* and the *corpus spongiosum*). At the same time the veins, which normally drain blood away from the penis, clamp down. Because blood flows in much faster than it can drain away, the pressure in the penis builds, expanding and firming up the chambers until the erection is complete. After orgasm, the nerves signal the system to work in reverse: the veins reopen, the blood drains out, the chambers deflate, and the penis returns to its flaccid state.

Each of these separate steps is required for a full and rigid erection. If something goes wrong, the result can be one of several different forms of erectile dysfunction: partial erection (inadequate for penetration), short-lived erection (not lasting long enough to be useful), or no erection at all.

IMPACT OF PROSTATE CANCER TREATMENT ON ERECTIONS

Loss of erections is often a gradual and natural function of aging. By age sixty-five, more than 25 percent of normal, healthy men have some degree of erectile dysfunction; the percentage rises with age. That means many men will become impotent whether they have treatment for prostate cancer or not. It also means that your age at the time of prostate treatment plays a big role in whether you will remain potent afterward.

One more point: In many cases, following treatment for prostate cancer, potency returns on its own over the course of time. The length of recovery varies. Many physicians advise their patients that it takes from six to twelve months. If erections do not return by that time, you may have to consider alternatives. Complete recovery may take as long as two years, but we know of men who were functioning well within six weeks after their operation.

With these thoughts in mind, let's look at the impact of the various prostate cancer treatments on sexual potency.

Watchful Waiting

Some men actually choose the most conservative prostate cancer treatment strategy, watchful waiting, because they don't want to risk impotence. Even this approach, however, can contribute to the problem. Left untreated, the tumor may grow to the point where it damages the nerves responsible for erections. If symptoms such as bone pain arise, interest in sex may disappear.

Sometimes, too, the problem is not physical but psychological. Some men who have untreated prostate cancer inside them become tense and anxious, and they may find it more difficult to perform sexually. Their mates aren't isolated from these feelings either. A wife may not feel comfortable initiating sex if she considers her husband ill or not interested. Or the man may avoid sex out of the erroneous belief that his cancer is "contagious."

In such cases, a little education can go a long way. Cancer is not a communicable disease. Should a prostate cell somehow be transmitted through ejaculation, it is biologically impossible for it to grow into a tumor inside another person's body. Counseling can also help relieve anxiety about cancer, which in turn can contribute to a more relaxed attitude about sex.

Surgery

If during surgery it is discovered that the cancer affects the neurovascular bundles, they must be removed during surgery. When possible, surgeons attempt to preserve them, particularly in the "nerve-sparing" form of radical prostatectomy.

The risk of impotence following surgery depends on four factors: the stage and grade of the tumor; whether one or both neurovascular bundles are removed; how old the patient is; and what the man's potency status was prior to the procedure. Over 95 percent of men treated with conventional radical prostatectomy (involving removal of both nerve bundles) are likely to experience some degree of erectile dysfunction. If the patient is young, the cancer is confined to the gland, and all nerves are left intact, the overall rate of impotence is about 32 percent. That number rises quickly, though, if only one neurovascular bundle is spared; for example, 50 percent of men over sixty and more than 75 percent of men over seventy will be impotent. Of course, men who are impotent before the operation will not become potent afterward.

Radiation

Many men undergo radiation therapy rather than surgery because they have other serious medical conditions that would increase the risk of an operative procedure. These conditions, including heart disease, high blood pressure, and diabetes, can weaken the blood circulation system, which in turn can have an impact on erectile function. Furthermore, men with these conditions often must take medications that interfere with sexual performance. As a result, many men who are good candidates for radiation therapy may already be experiencing some degree of erectile dysfunction before treatment begins. The risk is higher among men who are smokers.

Still, the rate of impotence following radiation is usually lower than it is with surgery. Different studies produce different results, but recent evidence suggests that radiation leads to impotence in under 50 percent of cases. Some experts argue that the number is closer to 35 percent following external-beam therapy and about half that following seed implantation.

While impotence is an immediate consequence of surgery, the problem takes longer to develop following radiation. A man may not develop erectile difficulties for up to six months after treatment with beams or implants.

Hormone Therapy

The goal of hormone therapy is to counteract the male hormones that fuel the growth and spread of prostate cancer. Unfortunately, the major male hormone, testosterone, is also largely responsible for regulating a man's sexual appetite, or *libido*. That's why one of the most pronounced side affects of hormone therapy can be a virtually total lack of interest in sex. Since sexual activity depends to a large extent on one's psychological state, loss of libido leads to loss of performance.

One way to remove testosterone from the body is orchiectomy: removal of the testicles. Some men feel that without their testicles, they are no longer really men. Inability to achieve erection only adds to their burden. They may feel embarrassed to be intimate with their partners, ashamed of their disfigured and uncooperative bodies. Clearly these kinds of psychological concerns—sometimes called *body-image issues*—can deeply affect sexual interest and activity.

Perhaps 80 to 90 percent of men under sixty who have hormone therapy will not have enough libido and potency to achieve erections and engage in intercourse. Those taking single-agent therapy (such as DES) are less likely to become impotent; some sources place the number at around 20 percent. Unfortunately, this treatment approach is less likely to curb prostate cancer than combination hormone therapy.

Cryosurgery

This approach, described in detail in chapter 11, is such a new procedure that it's hard to judge its impact on sexual performance. Generally, the risk of impotence appears to be comparable to standard prostatectomy: Up to 80 percent of cryosurgery patients are left impotent because the procedure damages the erectile nerves. On the other hand, some experts believe nerve tissue that is frozen during the procedure but is unaffected by cancer may eventually heal. If this proves true, some men who had cryosurgery may enjoy a return of potency.

ASSESSMENT OF SEXUAL FUNCTIONING

If you are reading this book before your prostate cancer treatment begins, you can start preparing yourself for the possibility of sexual problems. Part of your treatment plan should involve a careful assessment of sexual functioning. One of your caregivers will question you about your sex life. To get the help you may need, it's essential you answer honestly.

Questions will focus on the status of your current relationship, how often you have sex, and how often you masturbate. You'll be asked about your erections in detail: how firm they are, how often they occur, whether you have them when you awaken in the morning. Make sure you report whether you experience any difficulty or pain during love-making or during orgasm. Some men have a degree of curvature in their erection; report this too, because it may have a bearing on your treatment and its outcome.

Uncomfortable as you may find this discussion, your caregivers need to get a clear idea of your sexual health before treatment begins. This way they'll have a good baseline with which to compare any problems you might have later, and can begin the process of selecting an approach for managing impotence should it occur.

BENEFITS OF COUNSELING

Counseling may be helpful for you and your mate. Many men find it difficult to talk about sexuality. If you and your partner haven't talked openly about sexual matters before, you may have your work cut out for you now. It's important that you try. Your mutual sexual happiness for the rest of your life may depend on it.

Counseling can help you and your partner identify, understand, and cope with the things you're worried about. You might even be given exercises you can do at home to reduce stress relating to sexual matters. You may find a little counseling can make it easier to come to decisions you're comfortable with.

A few examples make the point. We know a man who decided (without telling his wife) to spend $15,000 for a penile implant, thinking that it would please her. He presented her with his *fait accompli* only to find out that she was perfectly happy with—and even preferred—noncoital sex. She was turned off by what she called his "unnatural" erections, and so he underwent another procedure (and spent thousands of dollars more) to have the implant removed. In another case, a loving wife wondered why her husband of twenty-three years had stopped giving her hugs after his radiation therapy. The husband was afraid that she'd misinterpret any affection as a sexual overture and he wasn't ready to risk intimacy. Another woman lamented the fact that she had been married over thirty years, but her husband had stopped expressing physical affection in any form. "We've become brother and sister," she said, "because we have hit a topic we cannot discuss." These couples weren't very good at communicating. Had they undergone counseling, however, they might have learned ways to express their feelings and spared themselves emotional (and financial) misery.

CHOOSING YOUR TREATMENT

If you could distill the wisdom of every man who has walked this path before you, the advice would be simple: Learn about all your treatment options. As we'll describe in a moment, numerous techniques are available to give you good erections. No single option is best for every man, but there is probably an option that is best for *you*. Your mission is to find it. Include your partner or spouse in this process. Ideally, even the act of exploring this issue will serve to strengthen your bonds of intimacy.

Your choice of methods for sexual rehabilitation should match the style and pattern of sex you and your partner enjoy. A couple that is satisfied with intimacy a few times a year may not want to invest a lot of time and trouble—not to mention money—in an inflatable penile implant, while a more sexually active couple may consider it to be worth any investment.

A good strategy is to begin with the least invasive approach and proceed from there. You might, for example, try the vacuum device first. If this proves unsatisfactory, self-injection therapy or an implant are options to consider.

A word of caution: Make sure your expectations are realistic. Even with the ideal treatment, your erection will probably not feel the way it did before. The whole sexual process will be different, too—perhaps a little less spontaneous, requiring a little more effort, challenging your creativity and sense of exploration a little more. A realistic goal is to achieve erections that are sufficiently firm to allow penetration.

TREATMENT OPTIONS

Do Nothing

A significant number of men are impotent before undergoing treatment for prostate cancer. Others may be having difficulty with erections but can still have sex some or even most of the time. If you're in one of these categories, you may already have come to terms with your declining sexual potency.

If so, you may want to exercise the most obvious option: Do nothing. Nowhere is it written that you must pursue every possible avenue to potency. There is no rule that says you must have

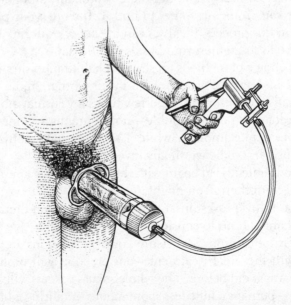

Figure 15.1: Vacuum device.

sex a certain number of times to qualify for manhood. Instead, you may simply want to relax about the issue and get on with your life. There's nothing wrong with that, as long as it's a choice you and your partner make together. Even though you may opt not to undergo treatment to restore erections, your penis is still sensitive. You don't have to engage in intercourse for you and your partner to enjoy sex and orgasms.

Psychological Counseling

A short course of counseling, either by itself or in conjunction with one of the other impotence therapies, can work by helping you adapt to the changes you're going through. For some men, guidance from a sensitive and concerned therapist may be enough to reduce anxiety and restore some degree of sexual function. Men using devices or medications for impotence may need ongoing support and advice that their physicians are unable to give. Often both the man and his mate benefit from such guidance, and it can be easier to talk to your partner with the guidance and support of an objective third party. Anything that enhances communication between you and your partner is worth pursuing at a time like this.

Vacuum Device

The vacuum device (Fig. 15.1) is a plastic cylinder attached to a pump. You insert your penis into the device and hold the cylinder tightly against your body. When the pump is activated (by hand or by batteries), a partial vacuum is created. The reduced air pressure draws blood into the penis. To maintain the erection, you slip an elastic ring, somewhat like a rubber band, around the base of your organ. This traps the blood and prevents it from leaving it after you remove the cylinder.

As a rule, the vacuum pump produces a workable erection in almost all men. Those who are able to use the device effectively are generally content with their choice. It's an economical method; the pump costs several hundred dollars and is usually covered by health plans, including Medicare. An unresolved question among experts is whether the pump facilitates or delays the return of natural erections. In any case, there are few, if any, long-term side effects. This is a reasonable and conservative approach for men who are likely to have natural erections return in time. "It works fine every time," said one man. "My wife and I signal our desire for sex by saying, 'Well, shall we go get pumped up?'"

The device has some disadvantages. Some men complain that the tension ring can produce discomfort at the base of the penis and can interfere with ejaculation. The pump is a mechanical device, and having to attach it and activate it tends to disrupt spontaneity. Men who have problems with manual dexterity might be unable to coordinate the process. Because blood does not flow into the penis while the ring is in place, the organ becomes cooler than

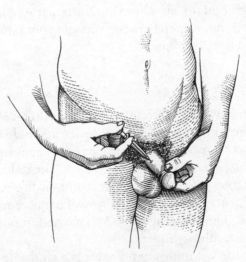

Figure 15.2: Injections as treatment for impotence.

normal. One special concern is that the tension ring must be taken off after thirty or forty minutes to restore the normal flow of blood.

A number of men stop using the device after a few months, some because their own erections have returned and others because they just don't like the device or have found success using another method.

Injections

In the mid-1980s, researchers discovered—virtually by accident— that injecting certain medications into the penis can stimulate erections. A decade later, injection (Fig. 15.2) is becoming the method that impotent men choose more often than any other option.

The first drugs available for this purpose were papaverine and phentolamine. When used by itself, papaverine can cause *fibrosis*—a kind of lumping or scarring of tissue at or near the injection site—in 5 to 10 percent of cases. Mixing this drug with phentolamine lowers the rate of this complication. More recently a substance called prostaglandin E1 has been found to be effective. Treatment that combines all three of these agents in a kind of "cocktail" may offer the best option for long-term use, providing an effective treatment for impotence with a decreased risk of side effects.

As recent studies have confirmed, injections are effective, resulting in erections in many patients. The needles used are tiny, so there is very little pain involved. Erections last between forty and sixty minutes. In some studies, two out of three men who used injections for a year said they would continue doing so because they were satisfied with the results and because they had experienced no serious complications. Another study found that 94 percent of men who had used injections for as long as seven years said they would continue indefinitely.

Still, the method is not for everyone. Men who have a fear of needles will probably never try it. One out of three men quits

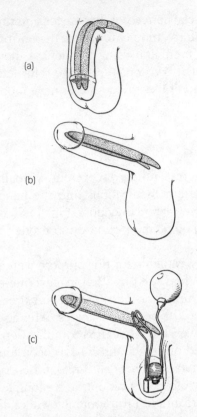

Figure 15.3: Penile implants: (a) malleable implant in normal and (b) erect position; (c) inflatable implant.

using injections for a variety of reasons: they find another treatment they like better, their erections return naturally, their partners are dissatisfied, they lose interest in the therapy, or they experience complications. Although prostaglandin E1 poses a lower risk of fibrosis, the risk remains. One study found that 10 percent of men who used the injections five times a month or more for seven years developed fibrosis. Between 10 and 20 percent experienced localized pain at the site of injection, but the pain was mild (2 on a scale of 10) and seldom lasted more than thirty seconds. Use of a preinjection analgesic minimizes the pain. In rare cases, use of penile injections can overstimulate the heart, leading to erratic heartbeat.

Implants

Penile implants replicate the function of the chambers in the penis that fill up with and hold blood during an erection. One implant is placed inside each corpus cavernosum in a surgical procedure that lasts anywhere from thirty minutes to two hours. Recovery from the operation takes about one to three weeks. There are different models available (Fig. 15.3).

SEMIRIGID OR MALLEABLE RODS

These rods, available in several lengths, afford the simplest approach to implants. A semirigid rod extends the penis and makes it permanently semierect. This is the simplest implant device, but some men find it a considerable inconvenience and difficult to conceal. The malleable rod is somewhat like a smooth, blunt pipe cleaner. When you want to have sex you bend your penis up into its "ready" position. When finished, you bend it down to its more relaxed profile. Up or down, your penis always will be the same length. The implant procedure is simple, and there is little risk of infection or other problems.

INFLATABLE IMPLANTS

The inflatable devices are designed to replicate several aspects of the penile hydraulic system. Consequently they are more complicated than the simple rods.

The *self-contained inflatable implant* has two cylinders, one placed inside each chamber, and a pump that is positioned behind the glans (head) of the penis. Squeezing the pump manually forces a liquid from a reservoir into the cylinders. When you no longer want to sustain the erection, you bend the penis, which causes the liquid to return to the reservoir.

The *fully inflatable implant* device has the pump tucked inside the scrotum. The pump is attached to a fluid-filled reservoir which is implanted in the abdomen. When you want an erection, you locate the pump and squeeze it gently. The fluid flows into the cylinders and enlarges the organ. Afterwards you release a little valve on the pump; the fluid returns to the reservoir, and the penis becomes flaccid.

Pumps are costlier and more complex than rods, and consequently so are the implant procedures. The different parts have to be inserted and connected, adding to the time on the operating table and to the time of postoperative recovery. Their advantage is that the erection is not permanent and is usually of a better quality. Still, some men might have trouble locating and activating the pump (the fully inflatable models are somewhat simpler than the self-contained implants). In some cases, the devices can malfunction, requiring reoperation.

Future Methods

Researchers are exploring ways to improve the treatment of impotence. One approach is to improve the ways of delivering medication. Perhaps the ideal method would be a cream that could be applied to the skin of the penis—no implants, no needles, no pumps. An automatic injection system would make it easier to inject drugs by using a button-activated spring rather than a syringe. Meanwhile, a device that inserts medication directly into the urethra may be available soon. And eventually new drugs will become available that produce results while being easier and safer to use.

VOICES OF EXPERIENCE

"You do not have to have intercourse and you do not have to have a good erection to have an orgasm," notes Art, age sixty-six. "There are other ways to show affection and to reach mutual satisfaction. For a man who can't get a good erection, tender care and stroking will work. So will mutual masturbation or oral sex. When a man is not erect, it takes more stimulation, loving, and understanding. But the orgasm is absolutely as satisfying. Maybe more so, because you know your mate is being so understanding of your needs, as you are of hers. If you speak to your urologist and talk to the men who have been there, you'll find out that, sexually speaking, life does not come to an end after prostate cancer."

"It's a matter of reorienting your thinking," noted Virgil, age forty-nine, a textile sales manager from New Jersey who counsels men with prostate cancer. "The fear is, 'Okay, I know my wife loves me but I can no longer get erections so she's going to find some guy who can and I'm going to lose her.' I tell guys, look, your wife's with you because she loves you—not just because your penis gets hard but for all the other things you are and that you've brought to the relationship. And you've got to be able to trust her. Unfortunately, we live in a society that says if you're not doing it in the missionary position you're doing something kinky. We have to say it's all right to use your fingers, your tongue, your toes, some toys—whatever works to make both of you happy. And it's a matter of educating the man about ways to experience a new kind of pleasure until—and if—the erection returns."

"I couldn't care less about the impotence," said Lois, wife of a prostate cancer survivor in Oregon. "Just knowing my husband is alive and sleeping next to me means more to me than a 'roll in the hay.' Of course I miss the sexual part of marriage, but I tell my husband 'I have a good memory.' I would love to have that part of our marriage back, but not at the cost of my husband's early death. Sex is not the most important thing to wives, but closeness is—holding hands, a peck on the cheek for no reason, the little things that are the natural actions between two people who love one another."

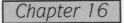

Chapter 16

Other Kinds of Support

Recovery from prostate cancer involves more than the healing of the body. Even when treatment is successful, the stress of managing a serious long-term illness can exact a heavy emotional toll on the patient and the family. A complete action plan takes into account the physical and psychological needs not just of the man with the diagnosis, but of those who love him as well.

This chapter discusses some of the resources available to you and your family, including support groups, counseling, and psychiatric therapies. The choice of when and whether to take advantage of these methods is yours. In our view, these methods promote healing and can contribute enormously to the quality of your life.

SUPPORT GROUPS

Too often, men confronting prostate cancer feel they have to tough it out alone. Perhaps they believe the myth that men are supposed to be stoic, that it is unmanly to feel—let alone express—fear or sadness or pain.

It need not—in fact, it should not—be that way. Acknowledging your feelings can be a positive and healing response to a stressful situation. Medical care is not the only form of treatment that can help you at times like this. To be complete, your action plan must take your feelings into account. One way to achieve that goal is to seek the support of others who understand your situation deeply and personally. You will find those men and women in a support group.

Different groups provide different kinds of support. Within the last decade a number of organizations have been formed that are devoted exclusively to meeting the needs of men with prostate cancer and their families. Examples include Man to Man, Side by Side, and US TOO. Other groups, such as the Wellness Community, serve a broader range of patients and achieve similar goals. Regardless of their structure, all groups serve people who share a common problem and a common need to find solutions. (To locate a group, see the resources section at the back of this book.)

Benefits of a Support Group

The benefits of a group can vary depending on the needs of the members and the leadership. Generally, though, groups can help you in the following ways.

TO SHOW YOU'RE NOT ALONE

Compounding the suffering of your serious illness is the feeling that no one else understands what you're going through. By virtue of its existence, a support group dispels that notion. Merely being in a room with other men confronting similar issues and wrestling with the same tough choices provides a powerful sense of reassurance and hope. When a healthy friend says, "I know how you feel," you might be tempted to respond, "You couldn't possibly." When another man with prostate cancer says the same thing, you know he means it.

TO UNDERSTAND PROSTATE CANCER AND THE TREATMENT OPTIONS AVAILABLE

On learning they have prostate cancer, many men try to read everything they can about what's happening to their bodies. It can be hard to make sense of the often technical, too often conflicting

ADVICE VERSUS INFORMATION

Responsible groups like Man to Man and US TOO explicitly forbid members to recommend treatment methods, medications, or physicians. Still, participants in support group meetings sometimes find it hard to resist giving advice. That's only human—but it's not always helpful.

There is a fine line between information and advice.

How do you tell the difference?

If it answers the question "What can I do?" it's information. If it answers the question "What *should* I do?" it's advice.

Remember that every case of prostate cancer is different. A suggestion that makes sense for an eighty-year-old widower may not be right for a fifty-two-year-old newlywed. If you attend a meeting where a well-meaning soul gives you well-meaning advice, thank him politely and take it with a grain of salt. If the advice is worthwhile, it will stand up to further discussion with your caregivers and with your family.

That's our advice—for your information.

information. It is even harder when information gets mixed up with advice (see box). Support groups, especially those that invite guest speakers, can be a rich source of answers and afford a great opportunity to separate the facts from the fantasies.

TO LEARN HOW TO LIVE WITH PROSTATE CANCER

Support groups bring you into contact with men who have been through the experience and who can prepare you for what may lie ahead. On a more practical level, members can exchange ideas for coping with cancer on a daily basis. Tips and strategies for dealing with prostate cancer or with the side effects of treatment can make a huge difference—not just in the quality of life, but perhaps in the quantity as well. A few years ago, researchers in California discovered that women with breast cancer who took part in support groups survived significantly longer than women who didn't attend. Supportive techniques promote stress reduction, which in turn can have an impact on the body's immune system and its ability to fight such cancers as melanoma and leukemia.

TO SORT OUT YOUR FEELINGS

Prostate cancer affects not just your body but your psychological state as well. It's natural to feel angry about what is happening to you, to feel anxious, afraid, or sad. Men often feel a powerful sense of loss related to their illness: loss of control, of youth, of independence, of wholeness. Depression is a common side effect of the diagnosis as well as of the treatment of prostate cancer. Support group members can help you explore other troubling feelings in a safe and sympathetic setting.

TO MASTER THE SITUATION

Many men with prostate cancer feel that the disease is making their lives spin out of control. Inside their bodies is a mysterious and potentially deadly growth that occasionally eludes even the most aggressive treatment. And patients must thread their way through the health care maze, dealing with physicians, hospitals, and insurance companies. Participating in group meetings can help restore your sense of mastery over your life. Leaders of US TOO groups usually begin their meetings with specific reminders: "Take control of your present and future health problems through education and regular consultations with your doctor. Take control of your health through diet, exercise, and stress reduction."

TO HELP OTHERS

At times, some men with prostate cancer may start to question the value of their life. They may feel vulnerable or "washed up." Participating in a support group, however, is a powerful antidote to that attitude. At no time do we feel more useful or valuable than when we are helping someone who needs our help. Your experiences, your awareness, your insight might be just the boost the fellow sitting next to you needs to make it over the next hurdle.

TO DEVELOP A REALISTIC PERSPECTIVE
Sometimes the most effective ingredient in a complete medical treatment program is a sense of hope coupled with a firm grip on reality. Taking part in a support group is an opportunity to see that there are other men with prostate cancer who have come to terms with their situation. The take-home message: You—like the other men in the group—have the power to manage your cancer and still lead a full and satisfying life.

What Happens in a Group Meeting

Each group has its own personality. The best way to understand what takes place during a session is to attend. There are usually two items on every agenda: listening and talking.

Many groups invite experts to visit and discuss topics of interest. Sometimes these talks are formal lectures, complete with slides and handouts; usually, though, they are informal, perhaps nothing more elaborate than question-and-answer sessions.

Groups often invite their own members to take the helm. A Connecticut group, for example, recently asked its resident computer guru to explain the Internet and demonstrate how to go online to find information about prostate cancer. Often, though, the group simply chooses a topic and has a free-flowing, roundtable discussion.

After a presentation, large groups often break into smaller work groups. These sessions allow more focused exchanges among members. Some men feel more comfortable expressing themselves in smaller groups.

Ideally, a group also offers opportunities for informal socializing. After the main program, many men linger over coffee and cookies to ask questions, share ideas, or simply talk about the home team's latest triumph.

Group Structures

The structure of the group depends on many factors: who sponsors it, who leads it, who can join, how often sessions take place, and what the goals of the organization are.

A sponsor can be any organization with an interest in helping men cope with their cancer. Typically, a hospital, religious organization, or community center makes space available in its facility and provides photocopying and other services. Organizations such as the American Cancer Society or the United Way frequently provide program materials or contribute funds to offset expenses. Having a sponsor usually means that the group offers its services free of charge. Sometimes, though, a group might take up voluntary collections to defray expenses.

Some groups are led by one or more health care professionals (usually nurses or social workers, but sometimes doctors) who take responsibility for organizing the group, planning programs, and conducting the meetings. Other groups—the ones people usually refer to as *self-help groups*—are peer-led, organized and run by the members. It is not unusual to find groups led by a team made up of one professional and one nonprofessional member. About half of the Man to Man groups around the country are led by members, the rest by professionals.

To meet the needs of their constituents, groups sometimes limit membership to a certain number of people or to those men who are at similar points in coping with their illness. For example, some groups include only newly diagnosed men or only those whose cancers are at more advanced stages. An offshoot of US TOO is a group called High Risers, whose members are coping with recurring cancer as indicated by rising PSA levels. People with special needs include those with severe sexual problems arising from treatment. This segment includes younger couples (especially those who have not finished raising a family), older men married to younger women, or newly married couples of any age. Some groups are devoted exclusively to helping couples work on these issues.

Groups that allow new members to join at any time are called *open groups*; *closed groups* restrict membership to those who are enrolled from the beginning. One goal of a closed group is to build a deeper sense of identity and cohesion among participants.

Certain groups are open to men only, while co-ed groups welcome wives (or other friends and relatives). The latter are an excellent source of strength and support for the partners of men with prostate cancer. Because so much focus is placed on the man in treatment, their partners' needs are often neglected. In some ways, women are "the other victims" of prostate cancer. Depending on the severity of the cancer and the type of treatment, the man may be suffering from mood changes, loss of sexuality, incontinence, and social withdrawal, all of which lower the quality of life for both partners. Both members of a couple may experience deep feelings of fear, depression, and anxiety. Participation in groups can help resolve some of those feelings. In our opinion, women should consider attending group meetings even if their mates are not interested.

US TOO meetings are open to wives, significant others, and family members. Most Man to Man groups approach things a little differently. Groups meet monthly, and the first meeting of each quarter is generally open to men and their spouses or caregivers. On subsequent months, in some Man to Man groups, men meet by themselves while the wives attend sessions at the same time but in another room. The women's organization is known aptly as Side by Side. Often the two groups then converge at the end of the session for a social hour. Having separate sessions allows individuals a greater freedom to discuss deeply personal problems with less risk of embarrassment.

Some groups, however, have discovered the value of focusing specifically on the needs of couples. For example, a group in New Jersey invites both the husband and the wife to all its regular meetings. Over the past few years, these couples have shared their most troubling problems and their deepest fears. "We started as strangers and have become good friends," said one member. "It took a few years, but gradually we reached a profound level of intimacy where we can discuss any issue that we're wrestling with. We've cried a lot, and we've laughed a lot too. We know we'll be there for each other. That is a powerful feeling."

Groups like Man to Man and US TOO are open-ended, which means they continue to meet as long as the members derive some benefit from being together. Some open-ended prostate cancer groups have been going strong for more than seven years. Time-limited groups, in contrast, have a set number of meetings, for example eight sessions over the course of four months. Such groups usually focus on a specific topic, such as dealing with sexual impotence.

Group Goals

The goals of the group also determine how it is structured and run. A therapy group, by definition, requires the leadership of a trained professional skilled in managing, identifying, and solving problems in a group setting. A support group or self-help group is less formal and less likely to focus on a single topic.

Some groups are strictly educational in their purpose. Members come to meetings, typically once a month, where they hear a presentation by an expert and discuss topics in a question-and-answer session. Over the course of a year or so, meetings will cover everything from the clinical aspects of cancer and its treatment to specific subjects such as nutrition, sexuality, incontinence, and use of medications. Among the speakers might be urologists, oncologists, pathologists, radiotherapists, nurses, nutritionists, social workers, psychologists, sex therapists, and spiritual counselors. This structure suits some men perfectly: They get the facts they seek but are not expected to contribute to the discussion or share personal feelings.

Other groups work to build intimacy and rapport among members, which can only happen through dialogue, interaction, and the fostering of relationships. Which group you prefer to join depends on your personal needs and your coping style. Many men belong to several groups to take advantage of the different features each one offers.

Who Attends Meetings?

Most of the members of a prostate cancer support group are likely to be men who have been treated or who are currently being treated for their disease. If they are experiencing adverse effects, they may be looking for specific advice on how to cope with their situation. They may want to know about additional ways of managing their illness. Or they simply may want to meet other men in similar circumstances.

A certain percentage of members are men who have just received their diagnosis and are trying to collect all the information they can before making their treatment choice. Talking with men who have already been through this process can be extremely valuable, and many support groups function as networks for just this purpose. They make available the names and phone numbers of men who are willing to serve as "mentors" to newly diagnosed patients. If you're wondering what it's like to undergo a radical prostatectomy or a course of radiation therapy, the best person to speak to may be the fellow with firsthand experience.

Another type of man at the meeting is what we might call the *activist*—usually the organizer of the group or its leader. This is the fellow who knows that taking action against the cancer is one of the best and most effective ways of restoring a sense of control. Activists keep tabs on all the latest developments in the field and share them with other members. They channel their emotional and physical energies into this constructive and positive outlet. Without such men, there would be far fewer support groups in existence, and fewer men would be able to benefit from this resource.

AMONG THE MISSING

One segment of the population that tends to be *under*represented in support groups is the long-term survivor. Typically, men join the group seeking answers. Once they have completed treatment and have dealt with just about every situation they can imagine, they may drop out of the program. Conversely, men whose cancer recurs or who start experiencing symptoms may join (or rejoin) a group, hoping to find new information or discover other options. As a result, newcomers miss the opportunity to meet former members who are coping successfully with prostate cancer over the long term. Instead, the new member may get a skewed perspective that exaggerates the rate of treatment failures and the incidence of side effects.

In describing the problem, one man said, "Where would organizations like Alcoholics Anonymous be today if the 'successes' didn't stay around to help the new participants?"

If you join a group and you notice a high proportion of men with advanced cancer or severe symptoms, don't be discouraged. Be aware that some of the healthiest prostate cancer survivors may have "graduated" from the group . . . and that, in a way, their absence can be interpreted as a sign of how effective group participation can be.

SUPPORT FOR COUPLES

The Couple as the "Unit of Care"

The best treatment programs recognize that cancer has an impact on everyone in the family. Because prostate cancer tends to strike later in life, when children are grown and away from the house, concern usually focuses on the man with the illness and his spouse. In social work terms, the couple becomes the "unit of care." As the wife of one of our patients expressed it, "Women suffer from prostate cancer, too."

The word *spouse* comes from the Latin meaning "to pledge." Remember that when you married, you pledged each other that you would stick together in sickness and in health. Prostate cancer puts that vow to the test. More than ever, you need to work together as a team.

When a man becomes seriously ill, the relationship between him and his partner changes. Often, to a greater degree than ever before, this person takes on the role of listener, supporter, and helper. Depending on the treatment and its outcome, the partner may be called on to act as nurse, on duty around the clock. Often this person helps enormously merely by maintaining the normal household routine to the extent possible. Sometimes the partner contributes by helping the man avoid becoming isolated and withdrawn from family and friends. In the best cases, partners provide continuing perspective on the situation—not false optimism, but realistic hope coupled with practical action.

That job description would challenge even the most highly trained professional caregiver. It underscores the fact that the partners of men with prostate cancer have needs and problems that must be addressed if recovery is to be as complete as possible. Dealing with a loved one's illness can seriously disrupt normal routines. The impact on the caregiver's own social life is often profound, as that person takes on demanding new responsibilities, some of which can seem overwhelming at times. In many cases the caregiver becomes the patient's advocate, communicating with doctors and hospitals, researching the illness, dealing with insurance company problems. Coping with the adverse effects of a loved one's treatment, including impotence and incontinence, can affect everything from the couple's sense of closeness to their ability to get a good night's sleep. The partner may feel anxious and fearful about the future.

Therapy for Couples

Taking part in self-help groups can go a long way to relieve the stress. Some couples, though, may not feel comfortable working through deeply personal issues in the company of strangers. Even those who benefit from their support groups might need additional help in the form of professional counseling or therapy. If the man declines to take advantage of these services, the partner can consider going for help alone.

A therapist can help in a number of ways.

IMPROVING COMMUNICATION

Preserving and nurturing the relationship depends on effective communication between the partners. Over the years, a couple often falls into habitual ways of speaking with each other—a kind of shorthand that substitutes for real communication. To break old patterns, they may need to learn—and agree to abide by—a few simple rules (see box, p. 248). To learn these rules and how to implement them, couples often benefit from the presence of a trained professional, such as a counselor or a psychotherapist.

FOSTERING INTIMACY

For many men, a large part of their identity and self-worth is rooted in their ability to perform sexually. The impact of prostate cancer and its treatment can profoundly threaten that identity. A sense of shame and embarrassment, or a fear of failure, can cause a man to resist initiating physical closeness with his partner. An Oregon man who became impotent after hormone therapy told his wife he didn't want to be physically affectionate because "it wouldn't be fair" to her. He meant that because he would be unable to proceed to intercourse and orgasm, there was no point in being close.

Many women acknowledge that for them, intimacy means more than just sexual intercourse. If asked to choose, a significant number say they would rather have affection in the form of hugging and cuddling, especially if the trade-off means their husband will be around for more years of life together. Many say that having sex just doesn't matter that much. And while a woman might make such a remark as a well-meaning attempt to reassure her husband, he may perceive the comment as a denial of his feelings

STRATEGIES FOR MORE EFFECTIVE COMMUNICATION

• *Use "I" statements rather than "you" statements.* For example, "I sometimes feel you're too busy to listen to me," instead of "You never listen to what I'm telling you."

• *Make a direct statement to express your needs,* instead of asking indirect questions. For example, "I'd like something to eat," instead of "Are you hungry?"

• *Don't expect your partner to be a mind-reader.*

• *Avoid "gunnysacking"*—the habit of stuffing all your past conflicts into an imaginary bag and dragging them all out during an argument, whether they are relevant or not.

• *Reduce the emotional level of your exchanges.* Avoid anger, sarcasm, threats, yelling—all the roadblocks to healthy and productive communication.

and his needs. "The problem," a Florida woman observed astutely, "is that it matters very much *to him.*"

Another factor is the ongoing difficulty some men experience with treatments for impotence. Often a man tries one of the therapies, such as the vacuum pump, but gives up if he encounters a problem or feels unsatisfied in some way.

A therapist can help solve problems associated with impotence therapy or guide couples through emotional turmoil. In the case of the husband who felt there was "no point" in being physically intimate, a counselor helped the couple communicate better so they could understand each other's point of view more clearly. The specific problems they worked on were the issues of who would initiate physical contact and when such contact was appropriate and welcome. The husband also learned that intimacy did not always require sexual intercourse. As he later expressed it, "I guess enjoying two movements of a three-movement symphony is better than hearing no music at all."

PRACTICAL SUPPORT

The social services department of your hospital can refer you to community agencies and other organizations to help with everyday concerns, such as:

- Finding someone to help with domestic chores or transportation
- Providing in-home caregivers to give the partner a much-needed respite
- Locating sources of financial support

OTHER PROFESSIONAL HELP

For eighteen months after his orchiectomy, Larry felt his world getting darker and colder. "My libido was totally gone," he said. "My mood plummeted. Before the prostate cancer, I had been energetic and happy, very active and very much in love with my wife. After treatment, my marriage started going down the toilet, and my life was turning to sludge. I didn't see any reason to go on living."

One day Larry thought he was having a heart attack. Deep down he sensed this might be a graceful way to end his suffering, but his wife, April, refused to let him give up. She dragged him to a cardiologist. The heart attack turned out to be a false alarm, but the doctor suggested that Larry try a course of treatment with one of the new antidepressant medications. "And about six weeks later I felt as if I were waking up from the dead. That pill literally saved my life—and my marriage. That was four years ago. I've been on the medication ever since, and I've never looked back."

Larry experienced one of the most serious and undertreated potential complications of prostate cancer: depression. In many cases, depression results from an imbalance of the brain chemicals responsible for controlling mood. In cancer, this imbalance can arise because of a combination of factors: the disruption in body function caused by the tumor, the impact of treatment, and the emotional turmoil triggered by the diagnosis and the stress of coping with the illness. In its medical sense, depression is much more than the normal and appropriate reaction to a difficult or stressful event—more than just "the blues." Symptoms include a persistently sad or anxious mood, feelings of emptiness and isolation, loss of pleasure in daily activities, and feelings of failure, self-blame, and guilt. Thoughts slow to a crawl and turn bleak, marked by hopelessness, helplessness, and even suicidal ideas. Depressed people find it difficult to concentrate, remember, or make decisions. Depression causes physical symptoms as well, including low energy, fatigue, and insomnia. Many people with depression wake up too early in the morning and can't get back to sleep. They may experience changes in appetite or body weight, or feel restless, irritable, or agitated.

As a result of his personal experience, Larry invited a psychiatrist to discuss depression at a support group meeting. "A lot of the guys came to the meeting thinking that their moods were just something they had to put up with, that as long as they could swing a golf club they were fine. But the speaker explained what depression was and that it could be treated. By the end of the meeting they were saying, 'Now I understand what I'm really going through.' Men just aren't used to talking about their feelings. But they don't have to suffer. I'm living proof of that. Better living through chemistry is no disgrace."

As Larry discovered, depression can be treated effectively. Many experts recommend an approach that combines judicious use of medication with talk therapy aimed at correcting negative thought patterns.

Low mood is just one aspect of the emotional fallout from prostate cancer. Other disturbing feelings can be addressed through psychological or psychiatric care. Effective medications are available to treat severe stress, anxiety, panic, and sleep disturbances.

In many cases, talking with a psychiatrist, psychologist, or other therapist can help you sort out other feelings as well. Many couples dealing with prostate cancer experience a deep and debilitating anger. The source of the anger is the illness, but too often their anger is expressed toward family members or caregivers—or each other. Counseling can help you recognize anger and find safe and effective ways of venting it. The same is true of fear. People with cancer often fear what caregivers call the "5 D's": death, disability, disfigurement, dependence, and disruption. (We would add *depression* as the sixth item on the list.) These fears are not irrational, but giving in to them can interfere with your recovery. A therapist can help.

One other emotional issue that too often goes unaddressed is the need to grieve. In almost all cases, prostate cancer triggers profound feelings of loss. Besides the loss of a body part, there is emotional loss as well—loss of a sense of immortality, of invincibility, of youth, of virility. Worst, perhaps, is the sense of loss of control over one's body and one's life. An effective way of coping with these feelings is to understand the need to go through a process of grieving. Steps in the process include accepting the reality of loss, working through the pain, adjusting to the new reality, and moving past the problem. The entire process takes a long time—perhaps years. It is worth the effort, but getting started may require some gentle guidance from a caring and sensitive professional.

Getting psychiatric help is not, as many men in our society believe, a sign of weakness. Quite the opposite: It is a sign of strength that demonstrates your desire to regain control over your life.

VOICES OF EXPERIENCE

Luke, a sales manager for a California precision-instrument company, learned he had prostate cancer at the remarkably young age of forty. He and his wife Fawn, age thirty-eight, had been married just over two years and were looking forward to starting a family. Fawn took a very active role in helping Luke get the help he needed. "We looked around for a support group and found one that told us women were welcome," Fawn said. "I did go to one meeting, but the emphasis was very much on what the patient himself needed, not the wives. Also, the few women who were there were much older than I am. I felt I needed more support from people my own age, who were dealing with the same sorts of issues." Unable to find a group in their area, Luke and Fawn took the initiative and started their own.

Bob, a seventy-five-year-old furniture maker, urges men to "find a support group before you do anything. If I had done that first, and learned what I know now, I think I would have made a smarter choice of treatments."

Steve, a fifty-eight-year-old computer consultant, and his wife, Betsy, found they were more comfortable in a group that included survivors of many kinds of cancer. They made their support group a weekly habit. "It's incredibly helpful knowing you're not alone," he said. "You see people who are in remission for long periods of time, who are dealing with all sorts of issues and who are still smiling, still active . . . still alive. It sounds odd to say, but it kind of takes the pressure out of the disease, making it more an everyday thing instead of a constant overpowering feeling of 'Why me?' "

Richard, a seventy-four-year-old former teacher, discovered the need for a group when he tried to discuss his situation with his friends. "They'd rather talk about baseball or their cars," he said. "They let me know—either through their words or their body language—that they didn't want to hear about it. I said to my wife, 'Years ago lepers were the outcasts. Now it's us guys with prostate cancer.' " Together he and his wife, Ruth, joined Side by Side, which, he says, "has been a tremendous help to both of us. We met other couples who, like us, were trying to come to terms with impotence. Through them I learned how important it was to give my wife the attention she needs. Even though we can't have intercourse, there are lots of ways we can still stay close. Sometimes a hug is all it takes."

Resources for Men with Prostate Cancer and for Their Families

Organizations

American Cancer Society
1599 Clifton Road NE
Atlanta, GA 30329
800-ACS-2345 (800-227-2345)
Offers free literature on cancer topics, sponsors support groups and cancer recovery programs, funds scientific research and community education.

American Foundation for Urologic Disease
300 West Pratt Street, Suite 401
Baltimore, MD 21201-2463
800-242-2383
Education for patients and professionals about urologic conditions, including prostate cancer and impotence; information about clinical research. You can also request information about their Prostate Cancer Support Network by calling 1-800-828-7866.

American Health Information Management Association
Office of Legislative Affairs
919 North Michigan Avenue, Suite 1400
Chicago, IL 60611
312-787-2672
Assistance for problems relating to medical records.

American Psychiatric Association
Division of Public Affairs, Dept. ACS
1400 K Street, NW
Washington, DC 20005
202-682-6325
Patient-education pamphlets on depression, anxiety, and other serious emotional disorders and their treatments.

American Urological Association
1120 North Charles Street
Baltimore, MD 21201
410-223-4310
Information for patients and professionals; supports research and education about prostate cancer.

Canadian Cancer Society
10 Alcorn Avenue, Suite 200
Toronto, Ontario
Canada M4V 3B1
416-961-7223
Information, support, research.

Cancer Care, Inc.
1180 Avenue of the Americas
New York, NY 10036
800-813-HOPE (800-813-4673)
212-221-3300
Information, counseling, and social services for patients and families. Also Prostate Cancer Education Council.

Cancer Hot Line
R. A. Bloch Cancer Foundation, Inc.
4410 Main Street
Kansas City, MO 64111
816-WE-BUILD (816-932-8453)
Books, referrals, information for cancer patients and their supporters.

Cancer Support Network
5895 Devereau Lane
Pittsburgh, PA 15232
412-661-8949
Support groups, educational programs, workshops for patients and families.

CaP CURE
1250 Fourth Street, Suite 360
Santa Monica, CA 90401
310-458-2873
Organization founded by financier Michael Milken, dedicated to finding a cure for prostate cancer.

College of American Pathologists
325 Waukegan Road
Northfield, IL 60093
800-323-4040
Professional organization of physicians specializing in pathology; provides information about developments in the prostate-specific antigen test.

Geddings Osbon Foundation
PO Box 1593
Augusta, GA 30903-1593
800-433-4215
Information about impotence treatments from a maker of vacuum pumps and implant devices.

Impotence Institute of America
10400 Little Patuxent Parkway, Suite 485
Columbia, MD
800-669-1603
Sponsors the Impotence Anonymous support groups; provides other information about the condition.

Man to Man
c/o American Cancer Society
1599 Clifton Rd, NE
Atlanta, GA 30329
800-ACS-2345 (800-227-2345)
Nationwide network of support groups for men with prostate cancer. Some groups also offer Side by Side, special groups or sessions for women partners.

The Mathews Foundation for Prostate Cancer Research
1010 Hurley Way, Suite 195
Sacramento, CA 95825
800-234-6284
Promotes public awareness of prostate cancer, funds research, offers telephone counseling, books, and videotapes.

National Association for Continence
PO Box 8310
Spartanburg, SC 29305
800-BLADDER (800-252-3337)
Information, a newsletter, resource guide, and physician referrals for people with incontinence.

National Cancer Institute
Cancer Information Service
National Institutes of Health Building 31, Room 10A24
Bethesda, MD 20892
800-4-CANCER (800-422-6237)
Government-sponsored service offering information about cancer treatments, research, and care centers; provides information for health professionals and their patients about all types of cancers.

National Chronic Pain Outreach Association
7979 Old Georgetown Road, Suite 100
Bethesda, MD 20814
301-652-4948
Free information packet about coping with pain.

National Coalition for Cancer Survivorship
1010 Wayne Avenue, 5th Floor
Silver Spring, MD 20910
301-650-8868
Network of survivors providing information about support groups; advocates for rights of cancer patients.

Patient Advocates for Advanced Cancer Treatments
1143 Parmelee, NW
Grand Rapids, MI 49504
616-453-1477
PAACT is a nonprofit organization especially active in promoting hormone treatments, cryosurgery, and other alternative therapies for prostate cancer.

Prostate Cancer Communication Resource, Inc.
PO Box 6023
Carefree, AZ 85377
602-488-1915
Nonprofit educational organization offering "Magic of the Mind," a dramatic presentation by Larry Becker, noted magician and mentalist and a prostate cancer survivor.

SIECUS (Sexuality Information and Education Council of the United States)
130 West 42nd Street, Suite 350
New York, NY 10036
212-819-9770
SIECUS provides literature on sexuality and illness.

Side by Side—*see* Man to Man

The Simon Foundation
PO Box 835
Wilmette, IL 60091
800-23-SIMON (800-237-4666)
Educational service focusing on treatment for incontinence.

Theragenics Corporation
5325 Oak Brook Parkway
Norcross, GA 30093
800-458-4372
Information about seed implantation, from a maker of radioactive materials.

US TOO International, Inc.
930 North York Road, Suite 50
Hinsdale, IL 60521-2993
800-80-US-TOO (800-808-7866)
Nationwide network of support groups for men with prostate cancer and BPH as well as their wives and families; provides information, counseling, and educational meetings.

Computer-Based Resources: World Wide Web

American Cancer Society
http://www.cancer.org

CaP CURE
http://www.secapl.com/prostate/capcure.html

CancerNet (National Cancer Institute)
http://wwwicic.nci.nih.gov/clinpdq/screening/Screening_for_prostate_cancer.html

Oncolink
http://cancer.med.upenn.edu/disease/prostate/index.html

Prostate Cancer InfoLink
http://www.comed.com/Prostate/

Prostate Pointers
http://rattler.cameron.edu/prostate/prostate.html

University of Michigan Prostate Cancer Home Page
http://www.cancer.med.umich.edu/prostcan/prostcan.html

Wellness Web
http://wellweb.com/PROSTATE/prostate.htm

Note: Bulletin boards and chat groups are available on the Internet and many online services, including Prodigy. PDQ files are available online from NCI and through CompuServe.

The Internet is expanding rapidly. Any list of sites on the World Wide Web is likely to be out of date as soon as it appears in print. To look for recent information, go to one of the Web indexes (such as Yahoo or Excite) and do a search for topics that interest you, whether general (prostate cancer, cancer support groups, radiation therapy) or very specific (PIN, TNM staging, etc.) There is a wealth of material available, both highly technical and for the layperson, and very often one site will offer links to many other related sites.

For Further Reading and Viewing

In addition to medical information, some of the following titles offer personal stories of men who have survived prostate cancer. Other books that discuss cancer and its treatment in general address topics relevant to men and their families who are coping with prostate cancer. Ask at your local library or bookstore for recommendations.

Altman, Roberta. *The Prostate Answer Book*. New York: Warner Books, 1993.

Gomella, Leonard G., and John J. Fried. *Recovering from Prostate Cancer: A Doctor's Guide for Patients and Their Loved Ones*. New York: HarperPaperbacks, 1993.

Kaltenbach, Don, and Tim Richards. *Prostate Cancer: A Survivor's Guide*. New Port Richey, Fla.: Seneca House Press, 1995.

Korda, Michael. *Man to Man: Surviving Prostate Cancer*. New York: Random House, 1996.

Lewis, James Jr., Ph.D. *How I Survived Prostate Cancer . . . And So Can You*. Westbury, N.Y.: Health Education Literary Publisher, 1994.

Lifelines: A Guide to Life with Prostate Cancer (videotape). Deerfield, Ill.: TAP Pharmaceuticals, Inc.

Marks, Sheldon, M.D. *Prostate and Cancer: A Family Guide to Diagnosis, Treatment, and Survival.* Tucson: Fisher Books, 1995.

Meyer, Sylvan, and Seymour C. Nash, M.D. *Prostate Cancer: Making Survival Decisions.* Chicago: The University of Chicago Press, 1994.

Morganstern, S., and A. Abrahams. *The Prostate Source Book: Everything You Need to Know.* Los Angeles: Lowell House, 1993.

Payne, James E., M.D. *Me Too: A Doctor Survives Prostate Cancer.* Waco, Tex.: WRS Publishing, 1995.

Phillips, Robert H., Ph.D. *Coping with Prostate Cancer.* Garden City Park, N.Y.: Avery Publishing Group, 1994.

Rous, Stephen N., M.D. *The Prostate Book: Sound Advice on Symptoms and Treatment.* New York: W. W. Norton & Co., 1992.

Walsh, Patrick C., and Janet Farrar Worthington. *The Prostate: A Guide for Men and the Women Who Love Them.* Baltimore: The Johns Hopkins Press, 1995.

Glossary

5-alpha reductase Enzyme in prostate cells that converts testosterone to DHT. Drugs such as finasteride (Proscar) that prevent this conversion are called 5-alpha reductase inhibitors.

ablation Removal or destruction. *See* cryoablation; combination hormone therapy.

adenocarcinoma Cancer arising in glandular tissue, such as the prostate.

adjuvant therapy Treatment that supplements or enhances the main, or primary, therapy.

adrenal androgen Male hormone secreted by the adrenal glands; adrenal androgens account for about 5 percent of the androgens in the body.

adrenal gland Organ located above the kidney; the two adrenal glands produce many substances, including small amounts of androgens.

adverse effect Negative or unwanted outcome associated with treatment.

alpha-blocker A drug that relaxes smooth-muscle tissue.

analog A synthetic version of a naturally occurring substance.

anastomosis The site where two structures are surgically joined together, as the bladder neck and urethra after removal of the prostate.

androgen Any male hormone. The major androgen is testosterone.

androgen blockade Use of drugs to disrupt the actions of male hormones.

androgen-dependent   Descriptive of prostate cells, benign or malignant, that are stimulated by male hormones and suppressed by androgen blockade. In contrast, cells that are androgen-independent do not respond to hormone therapy.

anesthesia   Prevention of pain awareness during a medical procedure. This may involve general anesthesia, with total loss of consciousness; local anesthesia, the numbing of a small area by injection of anesthetic; or regional anesthesia, the numbing of an entire region of the body.

angiogenesis   Formation of new blood vessels. Some anticancer drugs work by blocking angiogenesis, thus preventing blood from reaching and nourishing the tumor.

antiandrogen   A drug, such as flutamide, that blocks the activity of androgens.

antibody   Immune system protein produced in response to the presence of an antigen or a foreign protein.

anticholinergic drug   Medication that prevents or diminishes certain neuromuscular events in smooth muscle, including the bladder muscle. Such drugs are sometimes used to relieve urinary incontinence.

anticoagulant   A drug that inhibits blood clot formation.

antigen   A substance that stimulates the body to make antibodies.

anus   End of the rectum, through which feces pass out of the body.

artificial sphincter   Inflatable cuff implanted around the upper urethra for treatment of urinary incontinence.

aspiration   Technique of removing cells by suction through a needle.

asymptomatic   Without symptoms.

autologous transfusion   Use of a person's own blood, donated previously, to replace blood lost during surgery.

benign   Noncancerous or nonmalignant.

benign prostatic hyperplasia (BPH)   Noncancerous enlargement of the prostate.

biopsy   Removal and study under a microscope of a tissue sample. Sextant biopsy: Removal of six samples, one each from the top, middle, and bottom of each side of the prostate.

bladder Muscular organ that stores and expels urine.

bone scan Diagnostic image of the skeleton; used for detecting spread of cancer.

BPH *See* benign prostatic hyperplasia

brachytherapy Radiation treatment in which radioactive pellets are inserted into the prostate; also called interstitial radiation therapy or seed implantation.

cancer Abnormal and uncontrolled growth of cells.

carcinoma Malignant tumor arising in the lining or covering of an organ.

castration Elimination of male hormones, whether through surgical removal of the testicles (orchiectomy) or through administration of drugs to inhibit androgen production.

catheter Tube inserted into the bladder to drain urine from the bladder. A suprapubic catheter is inserted directly into the bladder via a small abdominal incision; a urethral catheter is inserted via the urethra.

cGy Short for *centigray*, a unit of radiation equivalent to the older unit, the rad.

chemoprevention Use of drugs to prevent cancer development or growth.

chemotherapy Use of drugs to kill or control cancer cells.

clinical staging Doctor's estimate of the extent of cancer, based on diagnostic tests. *Compare* pathologic staging.

clinical trial Test on human subjects of existing, new, or experimental treatments.

combination hormone therapy Complete blockage of androgen production involving orchiectomy plus use of antiandrogens; also called total hormonal ablation, total androgen blockade, or total androgen ablation.

computed tomography Computer-generated cross-sectional images of a portion of the body. Also called CT scan or CAT scan.

corpora cavernosa and **corpus spongiosum**   Chambers in the penis that fill with blood during erection.

cryoablation (cryosurgery, cryotherapy)   Use of extreme cold to freeze the prostate and destroy cancer cells.

CT scan   Computed tomography scan.

curative treatment   Therapy aimed at producing a cure. *Compare* palliative treatment.

cystoscope   Telescopic instrument for inspecting the urethra and the bladder.

debulk   To surgically reduce the volume of cancer.

DES   Diethylstilbestrol, a synthetic form of estrogen.

DHT   *See* dihydrotestosterone.

diagnosis   Process or result of determining the cause of a medical problem.

differentiation   Comparison of cancer cell appearance with that of normal cells; poorly differentiated cells are indicative of high-grade cancer.

digital rectal examination   Diagnostic test for prostate cancer and rectal diseases during which the doctor inserts a gloved, lubricated finger into the rectum and feels the prostate gland.

dihydrotestosterone   Powerful form of male hormone produced by the action of a prostate enzyme on testosterone.

distant recurrence   *See* recurrence.

DNA   Deoxyribonucleic acid, the genetic material contained within the nucleus of a cell.

doubling time   Period of time needed for a tumor to double in size.

DRE   *See* digital rectal examination.

dysplastic   Term used for cells marked by *dysplasia*, an abnormality of development in size, shape, or organization of adult cells.

ejaculate   Verb: to release semen during orgasm; noun: semen.

epididymis   Chamber outside the testicle where sperm travel after forming and where they are stored until they mature; leads into the vas deferens.

epidural anesthesia Injection of anesthetic drugs into the space around the sac that encloses the spinal cord.

epithelial cell Prostate cell that secretes prostatic fluid.

erectile dysfunction Problem achieving or maintaining an erection.

estrogen Female sex hormone. In therapeutic doses, estrogen inhibits the production of testosterone in men.

external-beam radiation therapy Radiation treatment administered from outside the body. *Compare* brachytherapy.

false negative Test result implying a condition does not exist when in fact it does.

false positive Test result implying a condition exists when in fact it does not.

flow cytometry Technique for analyzing cancer cells according to their DNA content, or ploidy.

frequency The need to urinate often.

frozen section Pathology technique in which tissue is quickly frozen, cut into thin slices, and stained for examination under a microscope to determine the course of action during a surgical procedure.

general anesthesia *See* anesthesia.

gland Tissue that secretes hormones or other substances.

Gleason score A method of classifying the grade of prostate cancer cells on a scale of 2 to 10. A pathologist gives a grade of 1 to 5, depending on its degree of differentiation, to each of the two most common types of cancer patterns in a tissue sample; the sum of those numbers is the Gleason score.

grade Degree of malignancy based on microscopic analysis of cancer cells; *see* Gleason score.

growth factor Protein that stimulates cancer cell division and growth.

gynecomastia Breast enlargement, sometimes involving breast tenderness; a side effect of hormone therapy.

hesitancy Inability to start the urine stream promptly.

hormone   A chemical secreted by one organ that circulates to, and acts on, cells elsewhere in the body.

hormone-dependent   *See* androgen-dependent.

hormone therapy   Use of surgery or drugs to block hormone production or activity.

hot flash   Sudden rush of body heat causing reddening and sweating; a common side effect of some types of hormone therapy.

immune system   The body's natural defense against infections or other foreign substances.

implant   Verb: to place within; noun: a device placed inside the body. Treatment for prostate cancer may involve radioactive seed implants; treatment for impotence may involve penile implants; treatment for incontinence may involve implanting an artificial sphincter.

impotence   Inability to produce or sustain an erection sufficient for intercourse.

incision   Cut made during surgery.

incontinence   Loss of urinary control. Overflow incontinence is a condition in which the bladder is full, and only small amounts of urine dribble out continuously. Stress incontinence is the release of urine due to abdominal stress or strain (e.g., coughing, physical activity) resulting from loss of sphincter muscle control. Urge incontinence is the release of urine resulting from uncontrolled bladder muscle contractions.

internal radiation   Treatment involving implantation of a radioactive substance; *See* brachytherapy.

interstitial brachytherapy   Implanting radioactive seeds into body tissue; usually synonymous with internal radiation.

intramuscular   Injected into a muscle.

intravenous (IV)   Injected into a vein.

intravenous pyelogram (IVP)   X rays of the kidneys, ureters, and bladder involving use of radio-opaque contrast material injected intravenously.

investigational   Under study; often used to describe drugs used in clinical trials.

Kegel exercise   Pelvic muscle exercise to help restore urinary control. Also called Kegels.

laparoscopic lymphadenectomy   Use of telescopic instruments for surgical removal of lymph nodes through several small incisions in the abdomen.

LH   *See* luteinizing hormone.

LHRH   *See* luteinizing hormone–releasing hormone.

LHRH agonist   Synthetic hormone used therapeutically to affect testosterone production.

libido   Sex drive.

linear accelerator   Machine that creates the high-energy beam of radiation used in external-beam radiation therapy.

local   In a small or confined area. *Compare* regional; systemic.

local anesthesia   *See* anesthesia.

localized prostate cancer   Tumor confined to the prostate.

local recurrence   *See* recurrence.

luteinizing hormone (LH)   Pituitary hormone that stimulates the testicles to produce testosterone.

luteinizing hormone–releasing hormone (LHRH)   Hormone produced by the hypothalamus that triggers release of LH by the pituitary.

lycopene   Substance found in cooked tomatoes; some research indicates it may reduce the risk of prostate cancer.

lymphadenectomy   Removal and examination of lymph nodes by microscopic study, used to determine if cancer has spread; it is often done prior to radical prostatectomy. Also called lymph node dissection or staging pelvic lymphadenectomy.

lymphangiography   X ray evaluation of lymphatic vessels.

lymphatic system   Spaces and vessels between body tissues and organs through which lymph, a clear fluid, circulates; the lymphatic system removes bacteria and other materials from tissues. Metastasizing cancer cells often appear in lymph nodes.

magnetic resonance imaging (MRI)   Technique using strong magnetic fields to produce detailed images of internal body structures.

malignancy   Uncontrolled growth of cells.

malignant   Cancerous; having the potential to spread.

margin   Edge of the tissue removed during surgery. A negative (surgical) margin is a sign that no cancer was left behind. A positive (surgical) margin indicates that cancer cells are found at the outer edge of tissue removed during surgery and is usually a sign that some cancer remains in the body.

metastasis (plural, **metastases**; verb, **metastasize**)   Spread of cancer via blood or lymph to a site other than where the tumor arose. Metastatic cancer is cancer that has spread from one part to another part of the body.

microvessel density   The number of blood vessels that nourish a tumor.

MRI   Magnetic resonance imaging.

negative margin   *See* margin.

neoadjuvant therapy   Treatment given before primary therapy begins.

neoplasm   Abnormal mass of tissue formed when cells reproduce at an increased rate; a tumor.

neurovascular bundle   One of two groups of nerves and blood vessels that run alongside the prostate and facilitate penile erections. Removal of either bundle or both during prostate surgery, or damage from radiation therapy, can lead to impotence.

nocturia   Frequent nighttime urination.

oncologist   Doctor specializing in treating cancer. The term is often modified to reflect the physician's specific area of expertise: radiation oncologist, surgical oncologist, medical oncologist, etc.

oncology   Branch of medicine dealing with tumors.

orchiectomy   Surgical removal of the testicles; castration.

overflow incontinence   *See* incontinence.

palliative treatment Therapy aimed at relieving symptoms. *Compare* curative treatment.

PAP Prostatic acid phosphatase.

pathologic staging Estimation of extent of cancer, determined by direct study of tissue removed during surgery. *Compare* clinical staging.

pathologist Doctor who specializes in analyzing tissues, then communicating the diagnosis to the treating physician.

pelvis The part of the skeleton that forms a ring of bones in the lower abdomen and that supports the spine.

penile implant Device used to restore erections.

penile Relating to the penis.

perineal Relating to the perineum.

perineal prostatectomy Removal of the prostate through an incision in the perineum.

perineum Area between the anus and scrotum.

peripheral zone The largest region of a normal prostate, where most prostate cancers develop.

PIN (prostatic intraepithelial neoplasia) Literally, tumor formation within the epithelium of the prostate. When present in biopsies, high-grade PIN often indicates that cancer is present elsewhere in the prostate.

ploidy An estimate of the amount of DNA in cells. If abnormally low or high, ploidy reflects the genetic derangements commonly present in cancer cells.

positive margin *See* margin.

primary cancer Refers to the site where the cancer begins.

primary therapy The first, and usually the most important, treatment.

prognosis Probable course of cancer; prediction of the outcome of treatment.

progression Worsening or recurrence of cancer.

prostate A male sex gland that produces prostatic fluid.

prostatectomy Surgical removal of all or part of the prostate gland.

prostate-specific antigen (PSA) A protein produced by the prostate. Levels of PSA usually rise in men with prostate cancer. The PSA test, which measures the levels in blood serum, is used to detect prostate cancer and to monitor the results of treatment.

prostatic acid phosphatase (PAP) A prostate enzyme that is elevated in some patients with prostate cancer. A PAP test is a blood test that measures levels of the enzyme; it is sometimes used to determine whether cancer has spread.

prostatic urethra The part of the urethra that runs through the prostate.

prostatitis Noncancerous inflammation of the prostate.

prosthesis Device used to replace a nonfunctioning or missing part of the body.

PSA *See* prostate-specific antigen.

PSA density (PSAD) Measure of the ratio of PSA to the volume of the prostate as determined by transrectal ultrasound; used to evaluate aggressiveness of cancer.

PSA level Amount of PSA found in serum, as determined by PSA test.

PSA velocity (PSAV) Rate of change in PSA level over time.

rad Acronym for "radiation absorbed dose," a measurement of the amount of radiation absorbed by tissues. The term rad is being replaced by cGy.

radiation Energy carried by waves or a stream of particles.

radiation oncologist Physician specializing in using radiation to treat cancer.

radiation physicist Member of the radiotherapy team who makes sure the appropriate dose of radiation is delivered to the right place in the body.

radiation therapist Radiation oncologist.

radiation therapy Use of high-energy rays to destroy the DNA of cancer cells and thus interfere with their ability to reproduce.

radical prostatectomy Surgical removal of the entire prostate gland with seminal vesicles and neighboring tissues. A radical perineal prostatectomy is performed through an incision in the perineum; a radical retropubic prostatectomy is performed through an abdominal incision.

radiologist Doctor specializing in interpreting X rays and other radiologic images.

radiotherapy Radiation therapy.

receptor A protein molecule on the surface of a cell that interacts with specific chemicals, such as hormones or drugs.

rectum Lower part of the large intestine leading to the anus.

recurrence Return of cancer following treatment. A distant recurrence involves the appearance of one or more metastases remote from the original tumor site; a local recurrence is the return of the cancer at the site of origin; and a regional recurrence is a return of cancer in the general vicinity of the original tumor.

refractory No longer responsive to a certain therapy.

regional Involving a relatively large area. *Compare* local; systemic.

regression Reduction in the size of the tumor or the extent of the cancer.

remission Complete or partial disappearance of cancer; or period of time when the disease does not progress. May be temporary or permanent.

resectoscope Instrument used in transurethral resection of the prostate, allowing the surgeon direct inspection of the prostatic urethra and adjacent prostatic tissue.

response Outcome derived from treatment or reaction to a drug or therapy.

retention *See* urinary retention.

retropubic Behind the pubic bone; a surgical approach to the prostate through an incision in the lower abdomen, in which the abdominal muscles are separated and the bladder moved aside.

sampling error Inaccurate assessment of cancer status resulting from failure of the biopsy needle to reach tissue containing cancer cells.

scrotum Pouch that holds the testicles.

semen   Fluid released during orgasm, containing sperm and seminal fluids.

seminal vesicles   Glands at the base of the bladder that release fluid into the semen during orgasm.

sextant biopsy   *See* biopsy.

side effect   A secondary reaction to a medication or treatment, usually—but not always—unwanted. *Compare* adverse effect.

sign   Objective physical change resulting from an illness which can be observed by the patient or doctor.

simulation   Technique using X rays to "rehearse" radiation treatment for prostate cancer.

small-cell carcinoma   Rare form of prostate cancer affecting certain cells other than glandular cells.

sphincter, urethral   Muscle that squeezes the urethra shut and provides urinary control.

spinal cord compression   Any process that results in pressure on the spinal cord, the spinal nerve trunks, or both; can occur when prostate cancer metastasizes to the spine.

stage   Extent of the cancer.

staging   Assessment of the size and spread of the cancer. *See* clinical staging; pathologic staging; TNM; Whitmore-Jewett.

stress incontinence   *See* incontinence.

stricture, urethral   Scar tissue from urethral injury, resulting in narrowing of the urethral channel.

strontium-89   Injectable radioactive substance used to treat bone pain.

surgical margin   *See* margin.

symptom   Subjective condition that results from a disease or disorder; usually cannot be observed or measured by another person.

systemic   Throughout the body. *Compare* local.

template   Device used to help physicians place seeds during brachytherapy.

testes or **testicles**   Male sex organs, source of testosterone.

testosterone The primary male sex hormone.

three-dimensional conformal therapy Form of external-beam radiation therapy using a detailed map of the prostate to deliver the maximum dose of radiation to the affected area while minimizing risk to neighboring tissue.

TNM Staging system for prostate cancer; **T** indicates the extent of tumor; **N** the extent of lymph node involvement; and **M** whether metastases are present. *Compare* Whitmore-Jewett staging system.

total androgen blockade *See* combination hormone therapy.

trans Prefix meaning "through," e.g., transabdominal, through the abdomen; transperineal, through the perineum; transrectal, through the rectum; transurethral, through the urethra.

transition zone Innermost area of the prostate, surrounding the urethra.

transrectal ultrasound (TRUS) Imaging technique using sound waves from a probe inserted in the rectum to generate an image of the prostate.

transurethral resection of the prostate (TURP) Surgical removal of tissue obstructing the urethra, performed with telescopic instruments inserted in the urethra; a form of partial prostatectomy.

TRUS Transrectal ultrasound.

tumor Literally, any swelling or lump. A tumor that forms because of abnormal cell processes, such as cancer, is also called a neoplasm.

tumor volume Measure of the amount of cancer present.

TURP Transurethral resection of the prostate.

ultrasound Diagnostic imaging technique using sound waves to create an echo pattern that reveals the structure of organs and tissues.

ureter Tube carrying urine from each kidney to the bladder.

urethra Tube leading from the bladder to the outside of the body; in men, the urethra traverses the prostate and the penis and provides a drainage channel for urine and semen.

urge incontinence *See* incontinence.

urgency Need to urinate right away.

urinary retention Inability to expel urine due to blockage or bladder-muscle dysfunction.

urodynamic study Test to evaluate function of the bladder muscle and urethral sphincters.

urologist A doctor specializing in problems of the urinary and male reproductive systems, including prostate cancer.

vacuum pump A device that creates an erection by drawing blood into the penis; a ring placed at the base of the penis traps the blood and sustains the erection.

vas deferens One of two muscular tubes (the vasa deferentia) that carry sperm from the testicles into the urethra.

vasectomy Surgical contraceptive procedure in which the vasa deferentia are tied or blocked to prevent release of sperm.

watchful waiting Conservative treatment of prostate cancer involving careful monitoring. Also called expectant management or deferred therapy.

Whitmore-Jewett staging system Classification system for evaluating the extent of prostate cancer, using the categories A, B, C, and D; now largely replaced worldwide by the TNM system.

Index

Page numbers in *italics* refer to figures.

A

ABCD (Whitmore-Jewett) staging system, 63, 69–70
TNM staging system vs., 71
abnormal cells, normal vs., 19–22
ACTH (adrenocorticotropic hormone), 12, 155
acupuncture, 191
acute prostatitis, 31
addiction, 204
adenocarcinomas, 25
adrenalectomy, 197
adrenocorticotropic hormone (ACTH), 12, 155
age, as risk factor, 34–35
agonists, 158–60
alkaline phosphatase, 51*n*
alternative treatments, 175–91
American Board of Medical Specialists, 86
American Cancer Society, 27, 33, 35, 36, 49, 85, 91, 111, 183, 186, 187, 241, 255, 260
American Foundation for Urologic Disease, 255
American Health Information Management Association, 255

American Psychiatric Association, 256
American Urological Association, 256
analogs, 158
androgen ablation (blockade), *see* hormone therapy
androgen-deprivation therapy, *see* hormone therapy
androgens, 10–13, 152
function of, 11
androgen therapy, salvage, 201
anesthesia, 124–25
antiandrogens, steroid, 161
antiandrogen therapy, *see* hormone therapy
antibodies, monoclonal, 181
anticipatory management, 214
antioxidants, 189
apex, of prostate, 5
asymptomatic signals, 27
autologous blood donation, 120, 122

B

bacterial prostatitis, chronic, 31
benign prostatic hyperplasia (BPH), 9, 11, 29–30, 44, 54

About the Authors

DAVID BOSTWICK, M.D., a pathologist and professor of pathology at the Mayo Clinic in Rochester, Minnesota, has devoted more than seventeen years to the study of prostate cancer and its origins. Author of over two hundred scientific papers, he has also written four books for medical professionals and is founder and editor in chief of *The Journal of Urological Pathology*. An internationally known conference speaker, Dr. Bostwick serves on the Prostate Cancer Advisory Group of the American Cancer Society, whose focus is prostate cancer research, education, and diagnosis. He is also on the board of advisors of US TOO International, the prostate cancer survivor support group.

GREGORY MACLENNAN, M.D., is board certified in both urology and anatomic pathology. He practiced urologic surgery for eleven years in North Dakota and has treated many men with prostate cancer. More recently, he has shifted his focus to surgical pathology and cytopathology, and has published a number of scientific articles. He is now an assistant professor of pathology at Case Western Reserve University in Cleveland, Ohio.

THAYNE LARSON, M.D., who trained at the Mayo Clinic in Rochester, Minnesota, is now consultant in urology at the Mayo Clinic in Scottsdale, Arizona, and assistant professor at the Mayo Clinic in Rochester. In his nine years of practice he has treated hundreds of men with prostate cancer. He has also published numerous articles in medical journals and has spoken about prostate cancer to professional organizations and men's groups in the United States and abroad.